Case Presentations in Paediatrics

Titles in the series

Case Presentations in Accident and Emergency Medicine

Case Presentations in Arterial Disease

Case Presentations in Clinical Geriatric Medicine

Case Presentations in Endocrinólogy and Diabetics

Case Presentations in Gastrointestinal Disease

Case Presentations in General Surgery

Case Presentations in Heart Disease (Second Edition)

Case Presentations in Medical Ophthalmology

Case Presentations in Neurology

Case Presentations in Obstetrics and Gynaecology

Case Presentations in Otolaryngology

Case Presentations in Paediatrics

Case Presentations in Psychiatry

Case Presentations in Renal Medicine

Case Presentations in Respiratory Medicine

Titles in preparation

Case Presentations in Anaesthesia and Intensive Care

Case Presentations in Urology

Case Presentations in Paediatrics
Second Edition

Vanda Joss, MBBS, MRCP
Consultant Paediatrician, Milton Keynes General Hospital

Stephen Rose, MD, MRCP
Consultant Paediatrician, Birmingham Heartlands Hospital

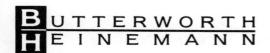

Butterworth-Heinemann
Linacre House, Jordan Hill, Oxford OX2 8EJ
A division of Reed Educational and Professional Publishing Ltd

A member of the Reed Elsevier plc group

OXFORD BOSTON JOHANNESBURG
MELBOURNE NEW DELHI SINGAPORE

First published 1983
Reprinted 1987
Second edition 1993
Reprinted 1993, 1996

British Library Cataloguing in Publication Data
A catalogue record for this book is available from the British Library.

Library of Congress Cataloging in Publication Data
A catalog record for this book is available from the Library of Congress.

ISBN 0 7506 1426 9

Typeset by Keytec Typesetters Ltd, Bridport, Dorset
Printed and bound in Great Britain by
Athenæum Press Ltd, Gateshead, Tyne & Wear

Preface

The introduction of greater comparability of junior to senior post numbers has improved the chances of advancing up the career ladder for those able to acquire regional recognition at registrar level. Choice of career is therefore made at the senior house officer level. Thus, in the UK, Membership of the Royal College of Physicians (MRCP) Part II will be necessary to enter the 'fast-track' lane, increasing the pressure to pass membership as early as possible with as few attempts as possible. We have written this second edition in the hope that it will help candidates over this particular hurdle as rapidly as possible.

The 'grey' cases in the written paper carry a significant proportion of marks, and for many they are the most difficult part. Each 'grey' case contains discrete pieces of relevant information, which can be in any part of the question and may be hidden among irrelevant or even misleading information. The cases published here follow this format, with (we hope) the same degree of cunning in spreading the relevant facts throughout the question. Some questions are more difficult than those in the examination, some easier, but the mixture will allow the reader to decipher the code of the questions. The topics of the questions do not reflect the frequency of disease; indeed, some cases are extremely rare, but sufficient information is contained in all questions to allow a logical conclusion while precluding an inspired guess. Several new questions are included in this edition which we feel improve the balance of the book and increase its scope. All questions have been carefully scrutinized; those not meeting exacting standards were either rewritten or discarded. All the answers have suffered the same fate and much updating was necessary, reflecting the rapid advances in medical technology. Similarly, the references have been completely revised and updated, with care taken to make sure quoted references are widely available.

The book continues to be aimed at those candidates taking paediatric membership, but is still of benefit to candidates of the adult membership because one of the four cases is usually paediatric. The Diploma of Child Health does not entirely follow the same format as Membership, but the approach of this book should also be useful to these cadidates. We hope our book will also be helpful to those studying for equivalent examinations outside the UK.

We would like to thank our publishers for the opportunity to publish this new edition and for their patience whilst awaiting the completed tome.

Vanda Joss
Stephen Rose

List of Abbreviations

ACAH	autoimmune chronic active hepatitis
ACTH	adrenocorticotrophic hormone
ADH	antidiuretic hormone
AIDS	acquired immune deficiency syndrome
ALL	acute lymphoblastic leukaemia
ALT	alanine transferase
AML	acute myeloblastic leukaemia
AMP	adenosine monophosphate
ANA	antinuclear antibody
ANF	atrial natriuretic factor
APTT	activated partial thromboplastin time
ARC	AIDS-related complex
ASOT	antistreptolysin O titre
AST	aspartate transferase
CAH	congenital adrenal hyperplasia
CGD	chronic granulomatous disease
CK	creatine kinase
CNS	central nervous system
CMV	cytomegalovirus
CPAP	continuous positive airways pressure
CSF	cerebrospinal fluid
CT	computed tomography
CVP	central venous pressure
DDAVP	desaminocys-d-arginine-8-vasopressin
DI	diabetes insipidus
DIC	disseminated intravascular coagulation
DISIDA	di-isopropyl imminodiacetate acid
DMSA	dimercaptosuccinic acid
EBV	Epstein–Barr virus
ECG	electrocardiogram
EEG	electroencephalogram
ELISA	enzyme-linked immunosorbent assay
EMG	electromyogram
ENT	ear, nose and throat
ESR	erythrocyte sedimentation rate
EUA	examination under anaesthesia
FAT	fluorescent antibody titre
FBC	full blood count
FEP	free erythrocyte protoporphyrin
Fio_2	ambient oxygen concentration

FSH	follicle-stimulating hormone
G6PD	glucose-6-phosphate dehydrogenase
GBS	Guillain–Barré syndrome
HAV	hepatitis A virus
HbAlC	glycosylated Hb
HBS Ag	hepatitis B surface antigen
HIV	human immunodeficiency virus
HLA	human leukocyte antigen
HMA	homomandelic acid
HOCM	hypertrophic obstructive cardiomyopathy
HUS	haemolytic uraemic syndrome
I : E	inspiration : expiration
IgG	immunoglobulin G
IPPV	intermittent positive pressure ventilation
ITP	idiopathic thrombocytopenic purpura
IVH	intraventricular haemorrhage
IVP	intravenous pyelogram
JCA	juvenile chronic arthritis
KCT	kaolin cephalin time
LH	luteinizing hormone
LHRH	luteinizing hormone-releasing hormone
LSCS	lower-segment caesarean section
MCH	mean cell Hb
MCHC	mean cell Hb concentration
MCV	mean cell volume
MMR	measles, mumps and rubella
MRI	magnetic resonance imaging
MSH	melanocyte stimulating hormone
MSU	midstream urine
NAD	nothing abnormal detected
NADP	nicotinamide adenine dinucleotide
NBT	nitroblue tetrazolium
OFC	occipitofrontal circumference
P_{CO_2}	partial pressure of carbon dioxide
PHA	phytohaemagglutination
Pi	protease inhibitor
PIP	peak inspiratory pressure
PNH	paroxysmal nocturnal haemoglobinuria
P_{O_2}	partial pressure of oxygen
PTA	proximal tubular acidosis
PTT	partial thromboplastin time
PUO	pyrexia of unknown origin
RBC	red blood cell

RF	rheumatoid factor
RSV	respiratory syncitial virus
RTA	renal tubular acidosis
RUL	right upper lobe
SBR	serum bilirubin
SCID	severe combined immune deficiency
SLE	systemic lupus erythematosus
SMA	spinal muscular atrophy
SSPE	subacute sclerosing panencephalitis
TBM	tuberculous meningitis
TORCH	toxoplasmosis, others, rubella, CMV, herpes
TRH	thyrotrophin-releasing hormone
TSH	thyroid-stimulating hormone
UKALL	United Kingdom Acute Lymphoblastic Leukaemia trails
VMA	vanillylmandelic acid
WBC	white blood count

1 Case presentations and questions

Case 1

A 6-year-old West Indian girl developed swelling of the left knee. She had been well that morning at nursery school, but then complained of pain in her left knee, which subsequently became swollen. There was no history of trauma whilst at nursery school that morning. There had been no recent illnesses, her appetite was good and she did not suffer from diarrhoea. She had had no previous hospital admissions.

Birth was by lower-segment caesarean section (LSCS) as the mother had had two previous LSCSs. The neonatal period was normal.

She sat at 7 months, began talking at 11 months and walked at 16 months. She was third-generation British and both parents were West Indian; her father, aged 37 years, was a bus driver and her mother, aged 34 years, was an office cleaner. The two older siblings were healthy. The family lived in a three-bed-roomed, semi-detached council house.

Examination

Height, 118.3 cm (90th centile).
Weight, 20.1 kg (50th centile).
Not clinically anaemic.
Pyrexial, 37.9 °C orally.
Pulse, 92 beats/min; blood pressure, 95/60 mmHg.
Short soft mid systolic ejection murmur.
Breath sounds normal.
Abdomen not tender.
No hepatosplenomegaly.
Bowel sounds normal.
Tonsils enlarged–not infected.
No rash.
Left knee–swollen, inflamed, tender, with restricted movement.

Investigations

Haemoglobin (Hb), 9.2 g/100 ml.
White blood count (WBC), 10.1 × 10⁹/litre.
Neutrophils, 73%; lymphocytes, 24%; monocytes, 2%.
Eosinophils, 1%; platelets, 215 × 10⁹/litre.
X-ray left knee, soft tissue swelling.

Questions

1. Give three possible diagnoses.
2. Give two further investigations.

Case 2

A 16-year-old boy is brought to you because of small stature. His parents are fairly sure that growth was much the same as his peers until 8 years of age. His general health has been good, appetite normal and, apart from morning headaches over the past few months, there have been no symptoms and no past history of note. He attends the local secondary school where he is of average ability, but he is not keen on sports.

The father is 178 cm tall and was pubertal about the age of 13 years. The mother is 152.4 cm tall; menarche was at 15 years. There is one 14-year-old male sibling, who is taller than his brother.

Examination

Height, 149 cm (<3rd centile).
Weight, 34.3 kg (<3rd centile).
No secondary sexual characteristics, infantile penis, both testes of prepubertal size.
All other systems normal.

Questions

1. What four important investigations would you do?

Case 3

An active and otherwise asymptomatic 8-year-old boy has a history of gradual onset of mild pain in the right hip preceded by a mild, febrile illness with coryza. The pain subsided in a few days but recurred 3 months later with aching in the right knee and groin associated with a runny nose and a low-grade fever. His paternal grandparents suffered from osteoarthritis and an aunt from mild rheumatoid arthritis. His siblings, a sister aged 6 and brother aged 11 years, were both well with no similar problems. His mother was pregnant and had just had a threatened miscarriage. His father was a French teacher and in good health.

Examination

Height, 117 cm (10th centile).
Weight, 19.3 cm (10th centile).
Pulse, 96 beats/min; sinus arrhythmia.
Blood pressure, 100/60 mmHg.
Heart sounds, normal–no added sounds.
Right hip: 10° internal rotation, 10° external rotation and 30° abduction.
All other joints, full painless movements.
Gait, limp on right leg.

Investigations

Hb, 11.8 g/100 ml.
Haematocrit, 36%.
WBC, 7.8 × 10^9/litre; polymorphs, 85%; lymphocytes, 15%.
Platelets 239 × 10^9/litre.
Erythrocyte sedimentation rate (ESR), 20 mm, in first hour.
Hb electrophoresis, AA.
Latex fixation, negative.
X-ray hips: sclerosis and partial collapse of the right femoral head with loss of the lateral superior quadrant, some cystic changes and slight lateral extrusion of the femoral head from the acetabulum.
Technetium-99 scan, focal decreased activity with surrounding zone of reaction and increased uptake in the right hip.
Bone age, 7 years.

4

1. What is the *most* likely diagnosis?
2. What two other conditions should be considered in the differential diagnosis?
3. What is the prognosis?

Case 4

A 10-year-old girl presented in the Accident and Emergency Department complaining of constant abdominal pain of 3 days' duration; there were no precipitating or exacerbating factors. Over the past few months she had been drinking up to 5 litres of fluid daily and waking several times during the night to drink. She was not enuretic and had no dysuria, vulval soreness, headaches or episodes of weakness. There had been no previous episodes or serious illnesses, but she had suffered a head injury recently which had not necessitated hospital admission.

Her adoptive father had recently left work with terminal Hodgkin's disease to be cared for at home. There were two older adopted siblings in the family. Academic progress at school was good although recently her teachers had reported a lack of concentration in class.

Examination

Examination revealed an apyrexial, well-nourished child, not clinically dehydrated, but complaining of thirst.
Height, 131 cm (25th centile).
Weight, 26.4 kg (25th centile).
Pulse, 80 beats/min; sinus arrhythmia.
Blood pressure, 110/60 mmHg.
Respirations, 24 breaths/min.
Tenderness in the umbilical area, right subcostal area and in both renal angles. No masses palpable.
Visual fields, normal to gross testing. Pupils equal and reacting to light.

Fundi normal.
No secondary sexual characteristics.

Investigations

Hb, 12.1 g/100 ml.
WBC, 5.4 × 10^9/litre.
Sodium, 134 mmol/litre.
Potassium, 4.4 mmol/litre.
Calcium, 2.1 mmol/litre.
Urinalysis, negative.
   After overnight fluid deprivation, the urine osmolality was 496 mosmol/litre, plasma osmolality 293 mosmol/litre.

Questions

1. Give three further relevant investigations.
2. What is the most likely diagnosis?

Case 5

A 3-year-old child presented in coma. He was born at term following a normal pregnancy. His initial development revealed that he had good head control at 10 weeks. By then he was able to smile. He sat with support at 8 months, and unsupported at 10 months, and walked at 16 months. He babbled and cooed at 8 months and he was able to reach out and grasp toys. He was able to say six words correctly at 18 months. He had not been taken to child welfare clinic and had not had vitamins at any time. He was artificially fed throughout and solids were introduced at 2 months. He regurgitated his food but this was not serious. He was not seen by a doctor for this symptom.
   His parents were poor and they lived with the child in an old house with an outside toilet. He was never immunized and the history revealed that he put everything into his mouth. His bowels were normal and his appetite recently had diminished. Over the previous 6 months, behavioural changes had been noticed.

On admission it was learnt that he had convulsed for approximately 45 min before stopping spontaneously.

Examination

Height, 84 cm (3rd centile).
Weight, 10.7 kg (3rd centile).
Pyrexial, 38 °C (axilla).
Pale, not clinically anaemic.
Pulse, 112 beats/min; blood pressure, 110/85 mmHg.
Heart sounds normal–no added sounds.
Responded to painful stimuli and simple commands.
Nuchal rigidity–positive Kernig's sign.
Pupils equal, reacted to light.
Fundoscopy, early bilateral papilloedema; no haemorrhages or exudates.
Diminished tone, upper and lower limbs.
Reflexes, sluggish.
Plantars, flexor.

Questions

1. What is the most likely diagnosis?
2. Give two differential diagnoses.
3. Give three investigations that you would do as soon as possible.

Case 6

A 3-month-old boy is admitted with a 24-hour history of lethargy and 12-hour history of crying, as if in pain, and vomiting. He had been a full-term normal delivery, birth weight 3.2 kg, breastfed with no previous history of note. There was one healthy 17-month-old male sibling and no significant family history.

On examination, his temperature was 39.3 °C and weight on the 90th centile; he was miserable but with no focal signs.

Investigations

Hb, 12.9 g/100 ml.
WBC, 14.9 × 10^9/litre; polymorphs, 51%; lymphocytes, 47%.
Sodium, 131 mmol/litre.
Potassium, 4.6 mmol/litre.
Urea, 4.3 mmol/litre.
Glucose, 7.2 mmol/litre.
Cerebrospinal fluid (CSF)–blood-stained sample: microscopy, RBC, 1000 × 10^6/litre; WBC, 5 × 10^6/litre lymphocytes, 0 neutrophils. Culture, no growth.
Glucose, 5.5 mmol/litre.
Protein, 2.3 g/litre.
Bag urine: micros; WBC, 1000 × 10^9/litre; culture, *Escherichia coli* > 100 000 organisms/ml, amoxycillin-resistant, co-trimoxazole-sensitive.
Blood culture, no growth.

He was started on amoxycillin prior to the sensitivity results, but 2 days later changed to co-trimoxazole. A repeat urine culture the same day yielded: micros; WBC, 20 × 10^9/litre; culture < 10 000 organisms/ml.

The temperature initially appeared to be settling, but after 2 days on co-trimoxazole it rose again to 39.5 °C and he was very irritable with vomiting. Again nothing could be found on examination apart from mild meningism.

Repeat septic screen: throat swab, scanty *E. coli*; nose swab, no growth; stool, no pathogens grown; blood culture, no growth.
Urine: micros; WBC, 5 × 10^9/litre; scanty RBC; scanty epithelial cells; culture, < 10 000 organisms/ml.
CSF: slightly turbid, cells; 27 × 10^6 lymphs/litre, 360 × 10^6 neuts/litre, 10 × 10^6 RBC/litre; smear, no organisms seen; culture, no growth; protein, 0.78 g/litre; sugar, 3.3 mmol/litre.
Blood sugar, 5.1 mmol/litre.
Urea electrolytes, normal.
Hb, 10.1 g/100 ml.
WBC, 18.3 × 10^9/litre; neutrophils 62%; lymphocytes 26%; monocytes 10%.
Film, toxic granulation.
Chest X-ray, normal.

He was treated for meningitis with penicillin and chloramphenicol, but the temperature continued to swing and 2 days later a large mass was felt on the right side of the abdomen. Repeat lumbar puncture confirmed improvement in the CSF cell count.

8

Questions

1. What two investigations would you do at this stage to aid diagnosis?
2. What is the most likely diagnosis?
3. What two lines of action would you take?

Case 7

A 10-year-old spina bifida boy was admitted from Outpatients with a pathological fracture of his left femur.

He had had an open lumbar myelomeningocele closed on day one. A muscle chart at this time demonstrated absent lower limb muscle tone, tendon reflexes and anal reflex absent. Sequential head circumference measurements demonstrated rapid enlargement and a ventriculoperitoneal shunt was inserted at 4 months of age. The distal catheter was lengthened at 18 months and 5 years. At 8 years the proximal catheter was replaced with difficulty and he began to convulse postoperatively.

He was controlled immediately by a mannitol infusion, but began fitting again 3 days postoperatively, requiring long-term phenobarbitone therapy. He had been well since discharge.

Social history

His parents had been unable to cope with the demands of a handicapped child and had placed him at a Dr Barnardo's home at $2\frac{1}{2}$ years. He had not seen them since.

He attended the remedial class of the local junior school and was considered of below average intelligence.

Examination

Weight, 32.1 kg (90th centile).
Height, 134.4 cm (50th centile).
Pulse, 84 beats/min; blood pressure, 115/75 mmHg.
Heart sounds, normal.

Peripheral pulses, present.
Chest, thoracic scoliosis.
Breath sounds, normal.
No hepatosplenomegaly.
Palpable faeces, sigmoid colon.
Bladder, palpable.
Rectal examination, faeces to anal margin.
Occipitofrontal circumference (OFC), 55.2 cm.
Shunt, filled and emptied rapidly.
Tone, power, co-ordination, normal in upper limbs, absent in lower limbs.
Pupils, equal; fundi, normal.
Reflexes, normal in upper limbs, absent in lower limbs; no anal reflex.
Deformity and swelling of left thigh.

Investigations

Hb, 10.7 g/100 ml.
White cell count, 7.3 × 10⁹/litre.
Sodium, 131 mmol/litre.
Potassium, 4.1 mmol/litre.
Calcium, 2.2 mmol/litre.
Urea, 3.6 mmol/litre.
Phosphate, 0.97 mmol/litre.
Alkaline phosphatase, 875 iu/litre.
Intravenous pyelogram (IVP), sequential series demonstrating worsening hydronephrosis and dilated ureters.

Questions

1. What is the most likely cause of the diagnosis?
2. What is the treatment?

Case 8

A 12-year-old girl is admitted to hospital with burns on her legs, which she obtained while playing near a bonfire on November

5th. The burns were treated with dry dressings and started to heal. While in hospital it was noted that her behaviour was odd. Her concentration span was very poor; she would suddenly change her attention from one conversation and shout something to another patient. On one occasion she had been walking unsteadily across the ward and fell for no apparent reason. Another time she had fallen out of bed.

She was the third child in a family of four. All other siblings were alive and well; there was no family history of note. The parents had been divorced 18 months earlier; the patient had been distressed at this and still saw her father regularly. Her behaviour had been unpredictable since the summer and in view of this she had been sent to stay with an aunt and uncle for some weeks during the holiday. At school decreasing concentration had led to a deterioration in performance.

In the past she had had tonsillectomy aged 6 years and the usual childhood illnesses including mumps, measles and more recently chickenpox.

Examination

Chest, cardiovascular system and abdomen, normal.
Neurological examination hampered by patient's lack of concentration. Cranial nerves, intact.
Fundi, normal.
She would suddenly grimace and have jerky movements of the limbs or the whole body. While trying co-ordination tests, movement was slow, but there was no tremor, only occasional odd posturing of the limbs. Movements of limbs were full and tone difficult to assess, but possibly slightly increased in the legs; there was no cogwheeling. Reflexes were all brisk and equal with an extensor plantar on the right, equivocal on the left. Gait was jerky and somewhat unsteady with heel–toe walking, and Romberg's impossible.

Investigations

Hb, 12.3 mg/100 ml.
WBC, 6.7×10^9/litre; normal differential.
ESR, 26 mm.
Skull X-ray, normal.

Questions

1. What is the diagnosis?
2. What two further investigations would you do?

Case 9

An 18-month-old Ghanaian girl with known sickle cell disease was admitted to hospital with a pyrexia. She had had a temperature for 3 days, associated with a cough and occasional vomiting. She had always lived in England and her parents were unrelated. Mother was at teacher training college and left the child with a babyminder during the day. Father was studying engineering. The only regular medication the child took was folic acid.

Examination

Pale, miserable child–pyrexial, 38.3 °C (axilla).
No jaundice.
Pulse, 124 beats/min; blood pressure, 85/50 mmHg.
Soft systolic murmur, left sternal border.
Respiratory rate, 30 breaths/min.
Breath sounds, normal.
Fauces, inflamed.
Tonsillar nodes, palpable–small, non-tender.
Tympanic membranes, normal.
Liver, 1 cm below costal margin.
Spleen, tipped.
Central nervous system, normal.

Investigations

Hb, 8.3 g/100 ml.
WBC, 22.7 × 10^9/litre; neutrophils, 63%; lymphocytes, 31%; monocytes, 4%; eosinophils, 2%.
Urea, 5.4 mmol/litre.

Sodium, 139 mmol/litre; potassium, 3.7 mmol/litre; bicarbonate, 22 mmol/litre.
Throat-swab culture, normal mouth commensals.
Midstream urine (MSU): micros.
WBC 13/cmm; culture, < 10 000 organisms/ml.
Urinalysis, nothing abnormal detected (NAD).
Blood culture, no growth.
Chest X-ray, some consolidation in the right middle lobe.

She was treated with penicillin intramuscularly because of the vomiting and the temperature settled after 24 hours. Penicillin V was then substituted but she again became pyrexial. It was thought that she was not taking the medication properly from mother and intramuscular penicillin was thus restarted. Again the temperature settled, but on changing back to penicillin V she became pyrexial within 24 hours. She continued to sit on her mother's lap, and was very miserable, withdrawn and anorexic. No new physical signs could be found on examination.

Questions

1. What three investigations would you do immediately?
2. What is the most likely diagnosis?
3. What is the treatment?

Case 10

A 9-year-old boy is referred to the Gastroenterology Outpatients by his general practitioner for investigation of chronic diarrhoea of 7 weeks' duration. He had been treated with antibiotics and antidiarrhoeal agents to no avail and was now beginning to lose weight.

The diarrhoea started 2 weeks after a camping holiday in Guernsey and, since then, he had passed loose stools three or four times daily. The diarrhoea was not obviously exacerbated by any foodstuffs and was not accompanied by abdominal pain, tenesmus or pain on defecation. His appetite was still good. The stools were not frothy, flushed away easily and contained no blood or mucus. He had had no previous similar episodes and no one else in the family was affected.

On systems analysis he admitted to the occasional headache which was mild, frontal, had no aura and resolved rapidly. The only previous medical problem was an admission following a road traffic accident. His school reports were above average and he had been made class captain for that year. His older brother had been elected school captain. His father was a successful 46-year-old merchant banker; his mother was 35 years old and a part-time freelance journalist. They lived in a large, luxurious detached house in suburbia.

Examination

Pleasant, intelligent co-operative child.
Height, 133.2 cm (50th centile).
Weight, 24.2 kg (10th centile).
Pulse, 88 beats/min; blood pressure, 140/100 mmHg–checked twice.
Apex beat not displaced.
Heart sounds, normal.
Peripheral pulses, normal.
Abdomen not distended; no hepatosplenomegaly.
Rectal examination–empty rectum.
Genitalia–normal prepubertal.
Pupils reacted to light; fundi, discs normal.
Tone, power and co-ordination normal.
Reflexes normal.

Investigations

Hb, 12.3 g/100 ml.
Mean cell volume (MCV), 80 fl.
Mean cell haemoglobin (MCH), 29 pg.
Mean cell haemoglobin concentration (MCHC), 32 g/dl.
WBC, 7.5×10^9/litre; neutrophils, 54%; lymphocytes, 43%; monocytes, 2%; eosinophils, 1%.
Sodium, 138 mmol/litre.
Potassium, 3.2 mmol/litre.
Calcium, 2.46 mmol/litre.
Phosphate, 1.35 mmol/litre.
Bicarbonate, 24 mmol/litre.
Urea, 2.0 mmol/litre.

Stools for giardia and bacteriology, negative.
Barium enema, normal.
MSU × 3, negative culture.
IVP, normal.
Electrocardiogram (ECG), normal.

Whilst in hospital his blood pressure settled at 125/90 mmHg and his diarrhoea responded to antidiarrhoeal agents. He was discharged with a month's outpatient appointment.

At this appointment he was noted to have ptosis and meiosis of the left eye with loss of sweating on the ipsilateral side of his face.

Questions

1. What is the most likely diagnosis?
2. Give two further important investigations.

Case 11

An 11-year-old girl who has had nephrotic syndrome since the age of 20 months presents in relapse for the 12th time. She has always been steroid-responsive and had highly selective proteinuria with a normal serum complement. A renal biopsy at the age of 2 years was consistent with minimal-change disease. She had a 6-week course of cyclophosphamide when 4 years old and was then relapse-free for 4 years. Her last relapse had been 9 months previously and she had been off steroids for 3 months.

She had a history of proteinuria and oedema 5 days prior to this admission, but for the previous 24 hours she had had severe abdominal pain, vomiting and dizziness on standing up.

Examination

Height, 132.7 cm (10th centile).
Weight, 45.2 kg (75th centile).
Apyrexial.
Oedema of ankles and face.
Pulse, 92 beats/min–sinus arrhythmia; blood pressure, 85/60 mmHg.

Heart sounds, normal.
Chest clear.
Abdomen–not distended, diffusely tender, bowel sounds present.

Investigations

Hb, 12.6 g/100 ml.
WBC, 7.6 × 10^9/litre.
Sodium, 136 mmol/litre.
Potassium, 4.2 mmol/litre.
Bicarbonate, 21 mmol/litre.
Urea, 6.0 mmol/litre.
Total protein, 54 g/litre.
Albumin, 14 g/litre.
24-hour urine, 9.5 g protein per 24 hours.
Blood culture, throat swab–no growth.
   Following admission she continued to vomit copiously up to 11
times daily. She continued to drink and passed 300 ml urine per
day with heavy proteinuria but still felt faint although her abdominal pain improved. Three days later she complained of pain in
her legs. On examination she had lost 1.2 kg in weight; there was
still very minimal oedema; blood pressure was 100/80 mmHg. Her
peripheries were cool, especially her feet which were cold with
loss of fine touch sensation and movement. The calf and thigh
muscles were tender bilaterally. Peripheral pulses were present
but decreased at the wrist; the femorals were weak, but neither
popliteals nor dorsalis pedis pulses could be felt. Heart sounds
were normal and the chest clear. Her abdomen was a little
distended and tender.

Repeat investigations

Sodium, 133 mmol/litre.
Potassium, 5.1 mmol/litre.
Bicarbonate, 16 mmol/litre.
Urea, 19 mmol/litre.
Albumin, 5 g/litre.
Hb, 15 g/100 ml.
WBC, 27.0 × 10^9/litre.
Platelets, 179 × 10^9/litre.

Questions

1. What are the two most important pathologies to consider?
2. What three investigations would you do immediately?
3. What three lines of treatment would you start?

Case 12

An 8-year-old boy diagnosed as a diabetic 10 months previously has been controlled on a daily dose of 16 units Humulin I insulin. Initially control was satisfactory, but 3 months ago he developed morning glycosuria at more than 2%, associated with ketonuria. During the day there was usually 0–0.5% glycosuria. Both mother and child were very careful with his injection dose and sites, diet and urine tests. Over the last 3 months, the insulin dose had been gradually increased to 28 units with no improvement in control. The glycolysated Hb (Hb AIC) was low.

Questions

1. What is the most likely cause for the glycosuria and ketonuria?
2. What would be the most helpful investigation?
3. In what two ways would you alter management?

Case 13

A 31-year-old Danish woman was admitted in established labour after falling on ice during a Christmas shopping trip to London. By dates she was 36–37 weeks' gestation; fundal height correlated with this estimation. Eighteen hours later she was delivered of a healthy female infant weighing 2.62 kg. No resuscitation procedures were necessary. The infant was put to the breast and sucked immediately. The following day she was seen by the paediatric senior house officer, who noted genital abnormalities.

The pregnancy had been uneventful and the mother had taken analgesics only for the occasional headache. No other drugs had been prescribed. This was their second child; the first, a male, had died aged 2 weeks of gastroenteritis.

The father, aged 32 years, owned a campsite just outside Copenhagen; the mother helped with the administration. They lived in a spacious mobile house on the site.

Examination

Weight, 2.59 kg.
Pulse, 142 beats/min.
Heart sounds, normal.
Peripheral pulses, normal.
Respiratory rate, 42 breaths/min.
Breath sounds, normal.
Liver, 1 cm; no splenomegaly.
Bowel sounds, normal–patent anus.
Genitalia–enlarged clitoris, fused labial folds.

Questions

1. Give two further important examination details.
2. What is the single most important diagnosis? Why?
3. Give two relevant investigations to the above diagnosis.

Case 14

A girl, aged 4 years and 2 months, was rushed to Accident and Emergency by ambulance, unconscious and convulsing. The convulsions were controlled immediately by intravenous diazepam, but the child became apnoeic, requiring mechanical ventilation.

The mother reported that the child had been well that morning, eaten a hearty breakfast and was playing with a friend when she became drowsy and then unconscious. The ambulance was called immediately.

The child had been previously healthy, with no major illnesses or previous hospital admissions. The only drugs in the house were aspirin and paracetamol syrup, kept in a locked bathroom cabinet. The family lived in a modernized thatched cottage, with new plumbing, in a small village. The father, aged 34 years, was headmaster at the local school; the mother, aged 29 years, had not worked since the marriage. Previously she had been a nursing auxiliary. She said she had felt quite depressed since the birth of her second child, now aged 3 months.

Examination

Height, 95.2 cm (10th centile).
Weight, 13.7 kg (40th centile).
Temperature, 36.1 °C.
Pulse, 142 beats/min; blood pressure, 80/50 mmHg.
Heart sounds, normal.
No spontaneous respiratory movement.
Tympanic membranes, normal.
Throat and larynx normal at intubation.
No abdominal masses.
Pupils dilated, poorly responsive to light.
Deep tendon reflexes, sluggish.
Plantars, downgoing.

Investigations

Hb, 11.9 g/100 ml.
WBC, 5.7×10^9/litre.
Sodium, 131 mmol/litre.
Potassium, 3.9 mmol/litre.
Calcium, 2.38 mmol/litre.
Phosphate, 1.81 mmol/litre.
Urea, 3.1 mmol/litre.
Blood cultures × 3, negative.
CSF: 4 lymphs; 244 RBC $\times 10^6$/litre.
Salicylate level–none detected.
Blood lead, 0.9 μmol/litre.
Urinalysis, negative.
Amino acid screen, normal.
ECG, atrial tachycardia–no abnormal complexes.
Chest, X-ray clear.
   The child was weaned from the ventilator over the next 18

hours, and regained full consciousness 36 hours after admission. No neurological sequelae were detected and the patient was discharged 5 days later with no diagnosis. Electroencephalogram (EEG) 6 weeks later was normal, but in the follow-up outpatients she was noted to be drowsy, unco-ordinated and walking with a wide-based gait. She was re-admitted and over the subsequent 90 min developed jerking of her left arm and leg. She recovered over the next 14 hours and was discharged 2 days later; all investigations, including a computed tomography (CT) scan, were normal. Over the following 8 weeks she was admitted twice with a similar clinical picture; both times she recovered rapidly with no ill effects. She was then admitted deeply unconscious and fitting. Again mechanical ventilation was required; supraventricular tachycardia developed which rapidly proceeded to ventricular fibrillation; resuscitation was unsuccessful.

Post-mortem revealed no macroscopic abnormalities.

Questions

1. What vital investigation was omitted?

Case 15

A 13-year-old boy is admitted unconscious to hospital having been pulled out of a swimming pool. He had been well and attended school that morning. He had eaten school lunch normally and an hour later gone swimming with the rest of his class. His teacher was uncertain about what had happened. He had been seen diving into the pool and possibly collided with another pupil whilst swimming. He was next seen at the side of the pool; he got out, then fell back into it. After being pulled out of the pool he was sat up on the edge by friends, spluttered and momentarily shook all four limbs. An ambulance was called immediately.

He had been born by normal delivery at 42 weeks' gestation following induced labour. There were no perinatal problems. He had had mumps, scarlatina, chickenpox then shingles 4 years later. He had recently changed school, but was said to be doing well. His father had died 10 years ago from rheumatic heart disease; his mother was well, supporting the family working as a nurse. She occasionally felt depressed and had difficulty sleeping. There was one brother, aged 11 years, who had broken his arm the day before.

On arrival he was unconscious and responding well to pain but immediately started shaking both arms and legs in a fine tremor. There were no tonic or clonic movements. His head was arched back and he was said to go blue. A pharyngeal airway was inserted but 1 min later it was coughed up and his colour improved. Following this he became alternately restless and drowsy; he did not respond to commands.

Examination

Apyrexial.
No obvious signs of injury.
Pulse, 72 beats/min; regular; blood pressure 90/70 mmHg.
Heart sounds, normal.
Chest, no added sounds.
Abdomen, normal.
No meningism.
Pupils equal–reacted to light; fundoscopy, normal; eye movements, normal.
Cranial nerves, normal as far as tested.
All limbs moved equally.
Tone, increased but equal.
Reflexes, normal.
Plantars, flexor.

Investigations

Hb, 13.7 g/100 ml.
WBC, 10.4×10^9/litre; 52% neutrophils, 44% lymphocytes, 4% monocytes.
Film, normal.
Sodium, 117 mmol/litre.
Potassium, 5.0 mmol/litre.
Urea, 3.5 mmol/litre.
Osmolality, 289 mmol/litre.
Glucose, 5.4 mmol/litre.

Skull X-ray, NAD.
Chest X-ray, NAD.

Questions

1. What four diagnoses would you consider first?
2. What four further investigations would you carry out?

Case 16

A 5-month-old baby presents with a rash and pyrexia of 40.5 °C. He had had a mild upper respiratory tract infection and watery eyes 5 days before, followed by a macular erythematous rash on the forehead and trunk with a pyrexia of 37.5 °C. A diagnosis of rubella was made. The rash gradually spread to the limbs and cheeks. He had refused all bottle feeds that day, screamed when a bottle was put in his mouth and on handling, and had had six loose, green motions.

In the past there was no history of note; the parents were unmarried but living together in rented accommodation. He was their first child and appeared well-cared for.

Examination

Length, 64.8 cm (25th centile).
Weight, 7.3 kg (50th centile).
Chest cardiovascular system and abdomen, normal.
Pharynx slightly inflamed–mouth clean.
Tympanic membranes, normal.
Central nervous system (CNS), normal.
Rash–raised erythematous non-purpuric patches with central white and bluish discoloration on the limbs.
On both calves, few small vesicular lesions.
Face and neck–rash less florid.
Trunk–macular rash.
Marked conjunctivitis with photophobia.
Lips cracked and weeping.

Investigations

Hb, 11.3 g/100 ml.
WBC, 20.9 × 10^9/litre; 82% neutrophils, 16% lymphocytes.
Film–toxic granulation of neutrophils.
Urea, 2.2 mmol/litre.
Sodium, 133 mmol/litre.
Potassium, 4.0 mmol/litre.
Blood sugar, 6.0 mmol/litre.
Throat swab, no growth.
Blood culture, no growth.
Chest X-ray, normal.
CSF: WBC, 21 × 10^6/litre; lymphocytes, 18; neutrophils, 3; RBC
0 × 10^6/litre; Gram's stain, no organism seen; sugar, 3.4 mmol/
litre; protein, 0.26 g/litre.

Questions

1. What is the diagnosis?
2. What are the four most likely causative agents in this child?
3. What is the usual outcome?

Case 17

A boy, aged 2 years 7 months, is referred from a rural hospital for
further treatment of gastroenteritis. He had been admitted 2 days
previously, after a 3-day history of vomiting. Oral rehydration had
been unsuccessful and, despite intravenous therapy, the child
was severely dehydrated on admission. Detailed questioning of
the mother revealed that the child had complained of abdominal
pain initially and then began forceful vomiting. He had vomited
up to five times daily before admission and only slightly less
thereafter. The vomitus was bile-stained but not bloody. There
had been no accompanying diarrhoea and the child had had a
normal bowel action the day after admission.

There was a history of two similar episodes 4 and 9 months
previously, again with forceful vomiting, but not diarrhoea. The
episodes had lasted 3 and 2 days, respectively, and resolved
spontaneously.

The pregnancy had been full-term and uncomplicated with a home confinement, despite this being the first pregnancy. The child had been breastfed exclusively for 3 months and then weaned. He was fully immunized.

The father was a 26-year-old cowhand; the mother was 22 years old and helped in the farm dairy. They lived in a two-bedroomed tied cottage, with open-fire heating.

Examination

Length, 92.2 cm (25th centile).
Weight, 11.87 kg (10th centile).
No jaundice or anaemia.
The child was apyrexial, had poor tissue turgor and dry mouth.
Pulse, 124 beats/min–poor pulse volume; blood pressure, 80/50 mmHg.
No added cardiac sounds.
Respiratory rate, 36 beats/min; no added sounds.
Scaphoid abdomen; no hepatosplenomegaly.
Bowel sounds not increased; rectum empty, no blood.
Comatose, responding to handling and pain.
Pupils responded to light; fundi, normal.
Reflexes, sluggish.
Plantars, downgoing. The child was felt to be approximately 15% dehydrated.

Investigations

Hb, 15.2 g/100 ml.
WBC, 8.7×10^9/litre.
Sodium, 146 mmol/litre.
Potassium, 3.8 mmol/litre.
Glucose, 7.3 mmol/litre.
Urea, 8.9 mmol/litre.
pH, 7.49.
Partial pressure of oxygen (Po_2), 12.1 kPa.
Partial pressure of carbon dioxide (Pco_2), 5.3 kPa.
Bicarbonate, 32 mmol/litre.
Base excess, +5 mmol/litre.
Standard bicarbonate, 29 mmol/litre.
Standard base excess, +7 mmol/litre.

Subsequent progress

Half the total of the child's estimated deficit was administered intravenously plus daily requirements as clear fluids over the subsequent 8 hours. The child regained consciousness and began to pass urine. Abdominal X-ray revealed a dilated stomach and duodenum, with little air distally. No intramural gas was seen.

Questions

1. What is the most likely diagnosis?
2. Give one further investigation.

Case 18

A 15-month-old girl is admitted with difficulty in moving her right arm and leg. She had had a mild cold during the previous few days, and on the day before admission the right leg was noticed to collapse under the child on two occasions. On waking up the following morning, she had paralysis of the right side of the body which regressed within a few hours. However, by midday a slight limp of the right leg was noticed. During the course of the afternoon, the parents noticed clonic right-sided seizures associated with mild drowsiness and recurrence of the right-sided paralysis. She had been a full-term, normal delivery, weighing 2.58 kg following a normal pregnancy. She sat at 6 months, walked at 12 months and spoke her first words before 1 year of age. She had had chickenpox and German measles without complications. There were no siblings and no family history of note.

Examination

Height, 77.2 cm (50th centile).
Weight, 10.9 kg (75th centile).
Pyrexial, 37.2 °C (axilla).
Fully conscious.
Subtotal, flaccid right-sided hemiplegia.

Right facial palsy, mainly affecting the lower part of the face.
All other cranial nerves intact.
Decreased right-sided reflexes.
Plantars: right, extensor; left, flexor.

Investigations

Hb, 11.3 g/100 ml.
WBC: 6.8 × 10⁹/litre; neutrophils, 56%; lymphocytes, 40%; eosino-
phils, 1%; monocytes, 3%.
Platelets, 246 × 10⁹/litre.
Prothrombin time, normal.
Blood culture, no growth.
Lumbar puncture–CSF: lymphocytes, 25; neutrophils, 5; RBC
0 × 10⁶/litre; RBC, 0; protein, 0.1 g/litre; sugar, 3.4 mmol/litre.
EEG: polymorphic delta activity over the left hemisphere max-
imum in the precentral area. Non-specific disturbances over the
right hemisphere.
Viral studies in stools, CSF and throat washings–negative.

Questions

1. What are the two most likely causes of her hemiplegia?
2. What three investigations would be most helpful at this stage?

Case 19

A 2½ year-old Caucasian girl presents with a 5-week history of
increasing pain in the left leg and difficulty walking upstairs. For
2 weeks she has had colicky, abdominal pain with screaming
episodes. Over the past 2 days she has developed a temperature
and been extremely miserable.

She is an only child, born at term by Kielland's forceps. She
was bottlefed and had no neonatal problems apart from mild
jaundice. Developmental milestones and growth had been
normal. She had been treated twice for otitis media by her
general practitioner and had had influenza 2 months previously at
the same time as her parents. She does not attend nursery school.

Immunizations were given at correct times. Her father is a bus driver; this is his second marriage, he had no children by his previous marriage. Her mother was a secretary in the civil service before the birth of her first child. Finances are a constant problem, even though they live in a two-bedroomed council flat.

On examination she was pyrexial, had some cervical lymphadenopathy, liver 2 cm below the costal margin and the spleen was palpable (2 cm). All joints appeared normal.

Investigations

Hb, 9.9 g/100 ml.
WBC, 10.0×10^9/litre; neutrophils, 1.2×10^9/litre.
Platelets, 153×10^9/litre.
ESR, 58 mm in first hour.
Alkaline phosphatase, 564 iu.
Serum alanine transferase (ALT), 26 iu.
Serum aspartate transferase (AST), 54 iu.

She was treated with aspirin, 100 mg/kg/day and following this her clinical condition improved, only to deteriorate again a few days later. She was noted to be pale and the repeat blood count was as follows:
Hb, 6 g/100 ml.
WBC, 3.7×10^9/litre; neutrophils, 0.2×10^9/litre.
Platelets, 22×10^9/litre.
ESR, 93 mm in first hour.

Questions

1. What are three differential diagnoses in order of priority?
2. What six investigations would you do to differentiate?

Case 20

A 17-year-old Spanish girl was admitted to the delivery room in established labour; her membranes had ruptured 14 hours previously. A normal male infant was delivered by breech, requiring no resuscitative procedures.

The mother had lived in England for the past 12 years and had not visited Spain for the past 2 years. She had not attended any antenatal clinics, was unsure of her dates and had smoked approximately 15 cigarettes a day during the pregnancy. The father was a West Indian, who worked as a porter in a meat market. Clinical assessment placed the gestational age of the infant at approximately 33 weeks. Birth weight was 1.23 kg, OFC 27 cm. He was nursed in an incubator and was noted to feed well from a bottle.

At 8 hours of life he suddenly had two apnoeic episodes. Examination after the first episode showed the following: pulse, 140 beats/min. No cyanosis, apyrexial, no jerky movements, fontanelle not bulging and he sucked well.

Investigations

Hb, 16.3 g/100 ml.
WBC, 10.2×10^9/litre; lymphocytes, 47%; neutrophils, 50%; monocytes, 3%.
Platelets, 100×10^9/litre.
Sodium, 138 mmol/litre.
Potassium, 3.8 mmol/litre.

Nothing abnormal was detected on further investigation, but despite feeding well and being very active he continued to have short apnoeic episodes.

Questions

1. Give three possible diagnoses.
2. Give four relevant investigations.
3. What is the most likely diagnosis?
4. Give two treatments for the recurrent apnoea.

Case 21

A 6-year-old boy is transferred for investigation with dyspnoea and an abscess on the anterior chest wall at the right sternal border second intercostal space. One month previously he had been admitted to a local hospital with fever, cervical lymphadenopathy, meningism, hepatosplenomegaly and right upper lobe (RUL) consolidation. Despite treatment with broad-spectrum antibiotics his condition had gradually worsened with increasing dyspnoea and finally the formation of an abscess.

He was a full-term, normal delivery, weighing 2.65 kg. There were no neonatal problems and at the age of 10 days he was adopted. He was next seen at the age of 5 months with bronchitis and loose stools. He improved on antibiotics. A sweat test was normal. At 6 months he was investigated for failure to thrive; nothing positive was found. He was placed on Complan and his weight increased. At 18 months he was not walking; no specific cause was found. His bone age was approximately 6 months. At 20 months he had lymphadenitis at the angle of the right mandibular ramus. This resolved spontaneously but at 2 years he had impetigo complicated by several small abscesses on the neck; no organisms were grown and he finally responded to antibiotics. One year later he had mumps. At $3\frac{1}{2}$ years he was found to be anaemic with hepatosplenomegaly. He was given a course of iron. At 4 years he got a chronic stye and following frequent antibiotic courses developed oral thrush. At the age of 5 years he had an anal abscess and again was noted to be small for his age. Investigations included an insulin tolerance test and jejunal biopsy. These findings were all within normal limits hence he was discharged.

Examination

Height 1 m.
Weight, 14 kg–both well below 3rd percentile.
Apyrexial.
Rash: erythematous discrete macular rash over trunk.
Pulse, 88 beats/min.
Blood pressure, 100/65 mmHg.
Heart sounds, soft systolic murmur left sternal edge.
Chest, dull to percussion right upper zone; bronchial breathing, right upper zone.
Abscess: 3 × 5 cm right chest wall; fluctuant, non-tender, not inflamed.

Abdomen: liver 4 cm enlarged; spleen, 5 cm enlarged, below costal margin.
Unable to walk, back painful and unable to sit without help.
Arms: normal movement, tone, power, sensation and reflexes.
Legs: both spastic, no voluntary movement on the left but 10° knee flexion just possible on the right. Sensation appeared intact for joint position, sense and touch. Reflexes all brisk and plantars both extensor with marked bilateral ankle clonus. Cranial nerves, intact.
Fundi, normal.

Investigations

Hb, 9.6 g/100 ml.
WBC, 18.9 × 10^9/litre; neutrophils, 76%; lymphocytes, 23%; monocytes, 1%.
Platelets, 425 × 10^9/litre.
IgA, 1.5 g/litre (normal, 0.3–1.5 g/litre).
IgG, 14.7 g/litre (normal, 5–14.0 g/litre).
IgM, 2.0 g/litre (normal, 0.5–2.0 g/litre).
Alkaline phosphatase, 448 iu/litre.
AST, 24 iu/litre.
ALT, 100 iu/litre.
CSF: WBC 0 × 10^6/litre; RBCs 165 × 10^6/litre.
Protein, 3 g/litre. Culture, sterile.
Abscess fluid drained, 15 ml; culture, *Aspergillus fumigatus*.
B and T cell numbers in peripheral blood, normal.
Phytohaemagglutinin (PHA) response within normal range.
C3/C4, normal.
Chest X-ray: consolidation right upper lobe; also patchy consolidation, right middle lobe.
Abdominal ultrasound: large liver and spleen, no ascites.
Bone marrow, hyperplasia of myelocytic line.
24-hour urinary vanillylmandelic acid (VMA), not raised.

Questions

1. What is the anatomical site of the neurological lesion?
2. What is the most likely diagnosis?
3. What four further investigations would you do?
4. What two steps in treatment would you consider?

Case 22

A 6½-year-old girl was referred urgently to Outpatients with vaginal bleeding of 4 days' duration.

The bleeding was bright red, not accompanied by any discharge and required three or four sanitary towels daily. There were no other symptoms. There was no history of recent trauma and the child denied introducing any foreign body into her vagina.

There were two older boys in the family, the mother had her menarche aged 13 years and had been sterilized after the birth of her third child.

The pregnancy had been normal, birth weight at term 3.21 kg, and there were no neonatal problems. Her development had been normal and she was of greater than average ability at school.

The parents had separated 3 years previously. The mother, aged 38 years, had remarried. The children lived with their mother and stepfather, an army captain, and stayed with their father, a successful oil executive, alternate weekends.

Examination

Height, 119.8 cm (75th centile).
Weight, 21.0 kg (50th centile).
Multiple café au lait spots.
Pulse, 76 beats/min; sinus arrhythmia.
Heart sounds, normal.
Blood pressure, 90/55 mmHg.
Abdomen, no masses.
Rectal examination, reflex anal dilatation negative, no masses.
No neurological abnormalities.
No secondary sexual characteristics.

Investigations

Hb, 11.3 g/100 ml.
WBC, 4.2×10^9/litre.
Urinalysis, NAD.
Bone age, 9–9½ years.

Examination under anaesthesia (EUA): no vaginal foreign body, no vulval trauma, no anal abnormalities, no abdominal masses—ovaries normal.

Questions

1. Give two possible diagnoses.
2. Give two further investigations to confirm the diagnosis.

Case 23

A 14-month-old boy has had a mild upper respiratory tract infection associated with occasional vomiting for the past 5 days, but for the previous 48 hours has had severe colicky abdominal pain with bloody diarrhoea and lethargy.

He was born at 36 weeks' gestation by caesarean section, weighing 2.7 kg, to a 21-year-old mother who now has another 3-month-old baby. His father is unemployed, and they live in a damp council flat. Apart from several upper respiratory infections and two episodes of otitis media, the child has been well, with his weight on the 25th centile. Developmental milestones have been normal.

Examination

Height, 72.2 cm (10th centile).
Weight, 9.3 kg (25th centile).
Pyrexial, 37.2 °C (axilla).
Pulse, 95 beats/min; blood pressure, 100/75 mmHg.
Heart sounds, normal.
Chest, clear.
Pharynx, inflamed, tympanic membranes dull.
Abdomen: diffuse tenderness, no rebound tenderness.
Rectal examination, normal.
Irritable and restless.
No meningism.
No central nervous system localizing signs.

Investigations

Hb, 7.9 g/100 ml.
WBC: 10.2×10^9/litre; neutrophils, 80%; lymphocytes, 15%; monocytes, 4%; eosinophils, 1%.
Platelets, 22×10^9/litre.
Prothrombin time, normal.
Partial thromboplastin time (PTT), normal.
Urea, 12 mmol/litre.
Creatinine, 150 mmol/litre.
Urinalysis: blood, moderate; protein, 2+.
Stool haematest, positive.

Questions

1. What is the most likely diagnosis?
2. Give three further complications.
3. What is the pathology on microscopy?

Case 24

A 4-year-old Irish girl is admitted with a 6-week history of occasional urinary incontinence both night and day, gradually increasing in frequency. She had an intermittent pyrexia and was generally a little 'off colour' in a non-specific way. There were no other urinary symptoms and no abdominal pain. She was a full-term normal delivery with subsequent normal development and was fully continent by the age of $2\frac{1}{2}$ years. Both parents were unemployed and there were three elder siblings, all in good health. They lived in a post-war prefabricated house which was so damp that water was running down the walls in two out of three bedrooms, and the family were therefore living in one bedroom and the sitting room; heating was inadequate. There was no family history of note except for the paternal grandfather, who had 'bronchitis'.

On examination her height and weight were on the 10th centile for her age and her general appearance was unkempt.

She was kept under observation for 1 week during which time she was noted to become more withdrawn and irritable. She liked to stay in bed or sleep for an increasing length of time each day, but when got out of bed she would run around in a jerky, tremulous fashion for a short period before retiring to bed again. She became more incontinent, more difficult to rouse, and continued to have a mild pyrexia. Apart from being drowsy and irritable there were no new physical signs.

Investigations

Hb, 11.3 g/100 ml.
WBC: 12.6×10^9/litre; neutrophils, 40%; lymphocytes, 53%; eosinophils, 4%; basophils, 3%.
Urea, 5.3 mmol/litre.
Electrolytes: sodium, 135 mmol/litre; potassium, 4.3 mmol/litre; bicarbonate, 24 mmol/litre.
Bilirubin, 17 mmol/litre.
Alkaline phosphatase, 562 iu/litre.
AST, 12 iu/litre.
ALT, 17 iu/litre.
Blood sugar, 6.2 mmol/litre.
Calcium, 2.1 mmol/litre.
Urine: micro., WBC, 3/cmm; culture, *Escherichia coli* $> 10^5$ organisms/ml (both results on two specimens).
Chest X-ray – enlargement of the right hilar shadow; lung fields, clear.

Questions

1. What is the most likely diagnosis?
2. What three investigations would you do to confirm it?
3. What are two of the most common complications?
4. What two other differential diagnoses should you consider?

Case 25

An 18-month Irish child was brought to the Paediatric Ward by a health visitor asking for a hospital opinion. The child had been walking 3 days previously, but had suddenly refused to walk and screamed whenever his left leg was touched or when the mother tried to dress or undress him.

His mother could recall no incident just prior to his refusal to walk. They lived in a second-floor flat, but the only internal step led to the bathroom which always had the door shut. His mother always carried him down the external stairs.

He was the only child; his mother was 20 years old, the pregnancy had been uneventful and he was delivered at term. Birth weight was 3.68 kg. He smiled at 7 weeks, sat at $6\frac{1}{2}$ months and started walking at 11 months. He could now use two-word sentences.

His father, aged 21 years, was a casual labourer with an irregular income. His mother helped to supplement this by office cleaning. They lived in a one-bedroomed, rented, private flat with shared bathroom. They were known to social services as they were often unable to pay the rent and the electricity supply had been disconnected twice. However, mother and child were reported as always being clean and well-dressed.

Two months previously the parents had answered an advert in a contact magazine and they had started to frequent wife-swapping parties. The husband had become involved with another woman and often spent nights with her. The wife had not been equally enamoured by the other husband and was distressed by these developments. A health visitor had then been asked to visit on a regular basis.

Examination

Height, 79.6 cm (25th centile).
Weight, 11.75 kg (50th centile).
Apyrexial.
Pulse, 98 beats/min; sinus arrhythmia; blood pressure, 80/45 mmHg.
Heart sounds, normal.
Chest, abdomen and neurological systems, normal.
Tender, warm swelling of left thigh.

Investigations

Hb, 12.1 g/100 ml.
WBC, 5.4×10^9/litre.

Blood cultures, negative.

X-ray: transverse fracture of mid third left femur; no new bone formation, normal cortex and trabecular pattern.

On further questioning mother recalled that the child climbed onto a dining room chair, his left leg slipped through the back and the chair then fell backwards on to his leg.

Questions

1. What is the maximum age of the fracture?
2. What is the most important subsequent investigation?

Case 26

A 4-year-old Arabian child was referred to Outpatients for a second opinion on the cause of his short stature. His mother stated that he had always been small for his age, but it was only over the last 9 months that she had noticed an increasing disparity in height against his peer group. His 3-year-old brother was now taller than him.

He was born at term, by spontaneous vaginal delivery in Saudi Arabia. Birth weight was unknown. He received a BCG immunization on day 2 and was discharged on day 4.

He had smiled at 7 weeks, sat at $7\frac{1}{2}$ months and walked at 15 months. He could now dress and undress himself, walk up and down stairs with one foot on each stair and could obey complex commands.

Three months prior to presentation he had developed a raised, non-itchy rash behind both ears and a month ago he had begun drinking more and was waking at night to drink.

He had had one hospital admission of 3 days for gastroenteritis.

His father was in the Saudi Arabian Army, his mother had never worked.

Examination

Height, 91 cm (<3rd centile); OFC, 48.0 cm (3rd centile).
Weight, 12.36 kg (<3rd centile).

Father's height, 175 cm (50th centile).
Mother's height, 152 cm (3rd centile).
Pulse, 88 beats/min; sinus arrhythmia; blood pressure, 90/60 mmHg.
No added cardiac sounds.
Chest, clear. Hepar, 3 cm.
Proptosis–he was unable to close his eyes completely.
Papular, non-itchy rash behind both ears.

Previous investigations

Hb, 11.9 g/100 ml.
WBC, 5.8 × 10^9/litre.
Chest X-ray, diffuse infiltration throughout.
MSU × 3, no growth.
IVP, normal.
Micturating cystogram, no reflux.

Further investigations

Hb, 11.3 g/100 ml.
WBC, 6.4 × 10^9/litre.
MSU, negative.
Thyroxine, 135 μmol/litre (normal range 75–150 μmol/litre).
Thyroid stimulating hormone (TSH), 1.7 iu/litre (normal range <1–5.8 iu/litre).
Serum osmolality, 296 mosmol/litre.
Urine specific gravity, 1008.
Urinalysis, negative.

Questions

1. What is the diagnosis?
2. Give two further important investigations.

Case 27

A female infant was born at 28 weeks' gestation, by dates, weighing 1.096 kg, the day after her mother had fallen heavily. There was no evidence of fetal distress during labour, she had a cephalic presentation and a controlled delivery. Apgar score at 1 min was 6 and at 5 min, 9. During the first hour of life she began to grunt on expiration which worsened over the next few hours. At 5 hours of life a chest X-ray showed a diffuse, uniform ground-glass appearance with air bronchograms extending beyond the border of the heart. An umbilical arterial catheter was inserted on the third attempt, and because of this antibiotics were commenced. Repeated blood gases demonstrated a falling pH and Po_2, and she was commenced on continuous positive airways pressure (CPAP) and finally on intermittent positive pressure ventilation (IPPV). A nasogastric tube was passed and aspirated 2-hourly, with minimal fluid recovered. On day 3 she was commenced on total parenteral nutrition. During IPPV the peak inspiratory pressure (PIP), rate, and ambient oxygen concentration (Fio_2) were 24 cmH$_2$O, 32/min and 0.75, respectively. On day 4 the ventilation settings were: rate 22/min; Fio_2, 0.45; pressure, 18 cmH$_2$O inspiratory pressure, 4 cmH$_2$O expiratory pressure; inspiration:expiration (I:E) ratio 1:1.5.

Blood gases: pH, 7.36; Pco_2, 5.21 kPa; Po_2, 8.5 kPa.
Bicarbonate, 21.3 mmol/litre.
Base deficit, 1.8 mmol/litre.
Standard bicarbonate, 22.1 mmol/litre.
Standard base deficit, 2.2 mmol/litre.

She was moving all limbs actively and was responding to being handled. She had a cyanotic episode with falling cardiac rate which did not respond to tactile stimulation, or hand ventilation 15 min after the above results. She was extubated and re-intubated. The removed endotracheal tube was patent and no haemorrhage from the larynx was seen on direct vision. After re-intubation her cardiac rate remained low at between 60 and 70 beats/min and she remained clinically cyanosed despite good air entry being heard.

Questions

1. Give two possible diagnoses.
2. Give one important investigation.

Case 28

A 10-month-old Cypriot boy was admitted with anaemia. Apart from two upper respiratory tract infections, he was well until 9 months of age, then developed a chest infection from which he made a good recovery. His general practitioner noted that he was pale and slightly icteric.

He was born at 42 weeks' gestation by normal delivery, birth weight 3.91 kg. Developmental milestones were normal. Both parents had lived in England for some years. There was one healthy female sibling, aged 7 years.

Examination

Length, 70.2 cm (10th centile).
Weight, 8.31 kg (10th centile).
Pale.
Pulse, 100 beats/min–regular; blood pressure, 90/60 mmHg.
Heart sounds, normal.
Chest, clear.
No abdominal organomegaly.
No neurological signs.

Investigations

Hb, 7.1 g/100 ml.
WBC; 11.0×10^9/litre; lymphocytes, 65%; neutrophils, 29%; eosinophils, 3%; monocytes, 3%; nucleated RBC, 3 per 100 WBC; reticulocytes, 3%.
Blood film comment: microcytes, poikilocytes and profound hypochromia; some RBC show basophilic stippling.
Hb electrophoresis, no abnormal bands detected.
Hb F, 72%; Hb A, 25%; Hb A_2, 3%.
Mother: Hb F, 2%; Hb A_2, 3.6%.
Father: Hb F, 5.9%; Hb A_2, 3.9%.

Questions

1. What is the diagnosis?
2. What test can be done for antenatal diagnosis?
3. What three long-term complications may arise?

Case 29

A 6-year-old boy was referred urgently by his general practitioner for headaches and vomiting.

Three days before referral the child had been playing in the garden and had fallen about 2.4 m (8 feet) from a tree. He had been winded, but had not hit his head, and within about half an hour had been climbing the same tree. However, 2 days later he complained of headache and vomited twice. On the morning of referral he still complained of a headache and continued vomiting. He also complained that he could not see properly and his mother noticed that he had developed a squint. He was then taken to the general practitioner.

He had developed otitis media after a mild coryzal illness 2 weeks previously. He had not been taken to the general practitioner until the drum burst spontaneously and the mother noticed the discharging pus. He was treated with erythromycin and the discharge cleared in 2 days.

The child was the fifth of seven and, as far as the mother could remember, had had an unremarkable birth, birth weight unknown, and had probably been fully immunized. He had not suffered any major illness and his siblings were generally healthy also.

His parents were from Nicaragua and had been in England for 8 years. The father had been unable to gain steady employment and the mother worked as an office cleaner, the children being looked after by the eldest daughter, aged 19 years. They lived in a three-bedroomed council flat.

Examination

Height, 118.2 cm (75th centile).
Weight, 20.9 kg (50th centile).
The child was irritable and miserable but apyrexial.
Pulse, 96 beats/min; sinus arrhythmia.
Chest clear.
Ears–both tympanic membranes normal, light reflex present, no retraction.
Throat not inflamed.
Abdominal system normal.

40

Nervous system: fully conscious and co-operative although irritable. Bilateral papilloedema, pupils equal, no photophobia.
Left sixth nerve palsy.
Tone and power equal.
Reflexes, normal.
Plantars, downgoing.
Kernig's sign, negative.
Mild nuchal rigidity.
Tripod sign, negative.

Investigations

Hb, 12.1 g/100 ml.
WBC, 7.3×10^9/litre; neutrophils, 73%; lymphocytes, 23%; basophils, 3%; monocytes, 1%.
Sodium, 131 mmol/litre.
Potassium, 4.3 mmol/litre.
Bicarbonate, 21 mmol/litre.
Urea, 2.1 mmol/litre.
Protein, 24 g/litre.

Questions

1. Give two further important investigations.
2. What is the most likely diagnosis?
3. What is the immediate treatment?
4. Give three other causes of this problem.

Case 30

A 4-year-old boy with known IgA deficiency is admitted for investigation of failure to gain weight for 1 year, his weight now being on the 10th centile, and his height having dropped from 75th to 50th centile.

He was a full-term, normal delivery, birth weight of 3 kg. He was breastfed for 1 week, then given a proprietary brand of baby milk. Developmental milestones were normal. He was first admitted aged 3 months with gastroenteritis and again at 4 months with a chest infection. Investigation showed all immunoglobulin levels to be low initially, but IgG and IgM levels were normal by 1 year of age; IgA level remained low. At the age of 2 years he developed constipation. This was initially treated with laxatives, enemas and an anal dilatation. For the past year, and especially recently, he has had episodes of diarrhoea and abdominal pain; the constipation has not been a problem. The stools are semi-formed, do not float, and become offensive during the episodes of diarrhoea. There is no blood or mucus. He has continued to have repeated upper respiratory tract infections including croup, not requiring admission to hospital. His appetite has been poor from the age of 1 year, he liked milk, drinking about 3 pints a day, but solids have always been a problem. His present appetite is worse than usual.

His grandfather has recently had infectious hepatitis. His sister also has IgA deficiency but with no clinical problems; his mother has hay fever. The family live in a three-bedroomed council house with garden.

Examination

Height, 101.3 cm.
Weight, 14.2 kg.
Pale, not clinically anaemic.
Pulse 84 beats/min; sinus arrhythmia.
Heart sounds, normal.
Chest, clear.
Pharynx, injected.
Tympanic membranes, normal.
Abdomen not distended, no hepatosplenomegaly.
Rectal examination, no faecal loading.
No buttock wasting.

Investigations

Hb, 11.4 g/100 ml.
WBC: 4.7×10^9/litre; neutrophils, 27%; lymphocytes 67%; eosinophils, 1%; monocytes, 5%. Platelets, normal.

Urea and electrolytes, normal.
Total protein, 76 g/litre.
Albumin, 35 g/litre.
Sweat sodium, 8 mmol/litre.
1 hour xylose level after 5 g dose, 1.69 mmol/litre.
Immunoglobulins: IgA, 0.3 g/litre (normal range 0.5–2.0 g/litre); salivary IgA, low.
Urine, NAD.
Stool: microscopy, no ova or parasites, no fat globules; culture, no pathogens isolated.
Throat swab, no growth.

Questions

1. What is the most likely diagnosis?
2. What two further investigations would you do to establish the diagnosis?

Case 31

Adrian was delivered vaginally at term after a normal pregnancy. Breastfeeding was initiated successfully; however, on day 4 he began to convulse. Lumbar puncture revealed a Gram-negative bacterial meningitis which was treated with parenteral antibiotics for 3 weeks. During the subsequent 4 months his head circumference increased from the 25th centile to greater than the 90th centile. A CT scan demonstrated dilated ventricles so an atrioventricular shunt was inserted. The shunt was revised uneventfully at 4 years of age.

At 5 years 9 months his mother reported in Outpatients that over the past 5 weeks he had become listless, anorexic and irritable. He became tired more rapidly and was not playing as actively with his friends. She thought he had lost weight. The general practitioner had prescribed a course of antibiotics for 10 days but without improvement.

Examination

Pale, irritable child.
Height, 106.3 cm (10th centile).
Weight, 19.4 kg (50th centile).
Temperature, 38.1 °C (oral).
Pulse, 96 beats/min; sinus arrhythmia.
Blood pressure, 110/70 mmHg.
Heart sounds, harsh pansystolic murmur, best heard left sternal edge.
No thrill.
Apex beat, sixth intercostal space mid clavicular line.
Peripheral pulses, present.
Respiratory rate, 32 breaths/min.
Trachea, central.
Breath sounds, clear.
Abdomen soft–no masses palpated.
No liver swelling.
Spleen, 3 cm.
Bowel sounds, normal.
Shunt, filled and emptied rapidly.
Pupils, equal and reacting.
Fundi, no papilloedema; scattered retinal haemorrhages.
Cranial nerves, intact.
Power, co-ordination and sensation–normal.
Reflexes, normal.
Plantars, flexor.

Investigations

Hb 9.7 g/100 ml.
WBC: 13.6×10^9/litre; neutrophils, 87%; lymphocytes, 9%; basophils 3%; eosinophils 1%.
Blood culture × 1 negative.
Chest X-ray, plethoric lung fields; heart–'boot-shaped'.

Questions

1. Where is the most likely anatomical position of the infective lesion?
2. What is the appropriate treatment?

Case 32

A 10-year-old boy presents with sudden onset of left-sided squint noted on waking up that morning. On closer questioning he admits to tingling of the upper lip on the left for 2–3 days but no other symptoms of note. Apart from childhood illnesses – measles, chickenpox and rubella – he has been well in the past. He had one episode of croup, aged 2 years, requiring admission to hospital. He has a sister aged 8 years. Their father works as a salesman and their mother as a secretary. They have all been well, but the maternal grandfather recently died from a stroke. At school he is average but making steady progress; he particularly likes sports and has many friends.

Examination

Height, 141 cm (75th centile).
Weight, 30.3 kg (50th centile).
Pupils, equal reaction to light; fundi, normal.
No meningism.
Minimal intention tremor on finger–nose testing on the left; no other signs of ataxia.
Marked left sixth nerve palsy.
Power, tone and sensation, equal and symmetrical.
Reflexes, normal.
General examination reveals no other abnormality.

Investigations

Hb, 13.6 g/100 ml.
WBC, 4.6×10^9/litre; normal differential.
Platelets, 302×10^9/litre.
ESR, 20 mm in first hour.
Urine analysis, NAD.
Skull X-rays, NAD.
CT scan, normal.
Audiometry, significant hearing loss on left.
   He is discharged home, but readmitted 2 days later with right-sided chest pain, over the lower two or three ribs, which is dull and constant in character. He has no cough and is apyrexial.

On examination there are no further physical signs; the left sixth nerve palsy is still present. The chest X-ray is clear. The pain lessens but does not disappear, and he is discharged again.

He is readmitted with urinary retention 2 weeks later. He is catheterized, but requires intermittent catheterization every few days for repeated retention. He also complains intermittently of headache and difficulty in walking.

Examination reveals variable neurological signs from day to day. Sometimes he has decreased power in both legs associated with brisk reflexes, ankle clonus and extensor plantars. During several of these episodes he refuses to try and walk. At other times neurological examination of his limbs is reported as normal. Cranial nerve signs remained unchanged, and general examination still reveals no abnormality.

A repeat CT scan is said to be normal.

Questions

1. What is the most likely explanation for this child's problems?
2. Give one pathological cause.

Case 33

A 15-month-old West Indian child presents with failure to thrive. He was a full-term normal delivery, weighing 3.14 kg; pregnancy was normal. He was breastfed from birth and solids were introduced at 4 months of age. He had been taken regularly to a baby clinic and received all immunizations. Clinic records revealed that his weight had been around the 50th centile until about 6–9 months. Since then he had gained very little weight and when seen, both height and weight were below the 3rd percentile; head circumference remained on the 50th centile. Mother had noticed swollen wrists at the age of 9 months. His general health was good, apart from several upper respiratory tract infections. His appetite was good, bowels open twice a day, and stools of normal form and colour. Developmentally he had smiled at 6 weeks, sat unsupported at 10 months, was not walking yet, but could say 'Mama' and 'Dada'.

There was one sister aged 3 years, and three step-sibs who were all well. They lived in a council flat, described by the health visitor as 'unsatisfactory and disorganized'.

Examination

Pale.
Pulse, 92 beats/min; blood pressure, 75/30 mmHg.
Heart sounds, normal.
Chest, clear.
No lymphadenopathy.
No abdominal abnormality.
Obvious swelling of wrists, ankles and costochondral junctions.
No muscle wasting or oedema.

Investigations

Hb, 9.9 g/100 ml; Hb electrophoresis, no abnormal bands.
MCV, 65 fl.
ESR, 4 mm in first hour.
Ferritin, 9 ng/ml (normal above 10 ng/ml).
Urea, 3.8 mmol/litre.
Sodium, 140 mmol/litre.
Potassium, 4.2 mmol/litre.
Bicarbonate, 14 mmol/litre.
Total proteins, 60 g/litre.
Albumin, 39 g/litre.
Calcium, 2.0 mmol/litre.
Phosphate, 0.8 mmol/litre.
pH: 7.38 plasma, 7.34 urine.
Alkaline phosphatase, 4800 u/litre.
AST, 8 iu/litre.
ALT, 15 iu/litre.
Xylose absorption test, 1.43 mmol/litre at 1 h.
Urinary amino acids, insignificant.
24-hour urinary phosphate, 3.8 mmol/litre (normal).
Acid loading test, urinary pH 5.28.
Stool microscopy, no ova or cysts seen, no fat globules; culture, no pathogens isolated.

MSU: microscopy, WBC 460 × 10⁹/litre; culture, *Escherichia coli* 10⁵ organism/ml.

MSU: microscopy, WBC 460×10^9/litre; culture, *Escherichia coli* 10^5 organism/ml.
IVP, minimal bilateral hydronephrosis and hydroureter.

Questions

1. What is the diagnosis?
2. What is the inheritance?
3. What is the treatment?

Case 34

A 5-month-old girl was referred from a district hospital for control of unprovoked temper tantrums and breath-holding attacks. The temper tantrums, episodes of tearless crying and breath-holding episodes had started 1 month previously. The parents were unable either to determine any provoking factors or to calm the child by any method so, in desperation, had taken her to the local hospital 2 weeks previously. The referring hospital had detected no physical or laboratory abnormalities except for two episodes of transient hypertension, thought to be secondary to her temper tantrums, and a short period of unexplained fever. Further questioning of the parents revealed that the child had been normal for the first 4 months. She was delivered vaginally at term, birth weight 2.63 kg, required no resuscitation and mother and child were discharged on day 7. She smiled at 7 weeks, was handling objects voluntarily at $3\frac{1}{2}$ months, had good head control and was able to raise herself on to her elbows. At about 4 months she started drooling, became more difficult to feed and began to vomit; this was thought to be due to the recent introduction of solids.

The parents were Jewish. The father was an accountant and the mother had been an actress until the birth of their second child. The family lived in a five-bedroomed flat. The three surviving siblings were healthy; one child had died aged 14 months, no diagnosis had been established.

This infant had had two previous chest infections and was recovering from a further episode.

Examination

Weight, 6.36 kg (25th centile).
Length, 63.2 cm (50th centile).
Head circumference, 42.8 cm (50th centile).
No jaundice or clinical anaemia.
Apyrexial.
Pulse, 132 beats/min; blood pressure, 95/60 mmHg.
Heart sounds, no added sounds.
No respiratory distress or recession.
Respiratory rate, 34 breaths/min.
Right-sided basal crepitations.
Tonsils, normal.
Tympanic membranes, normal.
Tongue, smooth, drooling.
Protuberant abdomen.
Liver, 1 cm.
No splenomegaly.
Bowel sounds, normal.
Irritable.
Right-sided corneal ulceration.
Pupils, equal.
Fundi, normal.
Tone and power equal in limbs.
Spontaneous movements all limbs.
Corneal reflex, absent.
Tendon reflexes, absent.

Investigations

Hb, 11.9 g/100 ml.
WBC, 1.3×10^9/litre.
Sodium, 139 mmol/litre.
Potassium, 4.2 mmol/litre.
Glucose, 5.1 mmol/litre.
Bicarbonate, 26 mmol/litre.
Urea, 1.9 mmol/litre.
Total protein, 69 g/litre.
Kaolin cephalin time (KCT)/ PTT, within normal limits.
Liver enzymes, normal limits.

Urinalysis: pH 6; no protein, blood or reducing substances detected.
Chest X-ray, patchy atelectasis right base.

Questions

1. Give two possible diagnoses.
2. Give two further important investigations.

Case 35

A 6-year-old girl is admitted 3 weeks after the onset of chickenpox. She had not been particularly unwell on appearance of the rash, but 4 days later started vomiting. The following day she developed colicky lower abdominal pain with diarrhoea which lasted for 5 days with occasional vomiting and anorexia. Over the next 10 days she only passed two loose motions, became intermittently pyrexial and after having some difficulty in passing urine, finally developed retention. The family are generally healthy, but her younger brother aged 4 years is just developing chickenpox. In the past there has been no significant illness or operation.

Examination

Distressed child.
Pyrexial, 40 °C (oral).
Pulse, 130 beats/min; blood pressure, 90/60 mmHg.
Heart sounds, normal.
Chest, healing chickenpox lesions.
Abdomen soft, no tenderness; bowel sound, present.
Mass, dull to percussion, extending from pubic symphysis to umbilicus.
Second mass, dull to percussion, about 7 cm in diameter arising from pelvis to right of midline deeper than first mass.
Rectal examination, hard faeces, marked tenderness anteriorly.
No neurological signs.

Questions

1. Give one important clinical procedure before further examination of patient.
2. What four important investigations would you do?
3. What is the most likely diagnosis?

Case 36

On Christmas Day a 13-year-old girl sampled her first wine; she later vomited. Two days later she developed a coryzal illness. Initially the nasal discharge was clear; it then became purulent and she complained of a frontal headache. The headaches persisted after the resolution of the coryza. She complained of frontal pain daily but still attended school. She did not complain of visual disturbances and was not nauseated. However, after 10 days of the frontal pain she complained of numbness of the left leg and collapsed on getting up from a chair. She was conscious on admission but became comatose over the following 4 hours.

She attended the local comprehensive school and was hoping to take several GCSEs.

She was the only child of the present marriage; the mother had a 19-year-old son by a previous marriage. The family lived in a three-bedroomed, centrally heated flat.

The patient had suffered no previous major illnesses.

Examination

Pulse, 132 beats/min; blood pressure, 110/65 mmHg.
Cardiac sounds, normal.
Respiratory rate, 24 breaths/min.
No added respiratory sounds.
Middle ear, not infected.
Semi-conscious–responded appropriately to simple commands.
Fundi: right, gross papilloedema; left, papilloedema.
Pupils: left, reacted to light; right, ptosis and pupillary dilatation.
Cranial nerves: corneal reflex intact bilaterally; right sixth nerve palsy; no facial asymmetry.

Gag reflex intact.
Reflexes, reduced on left.
Plantars: right, downgoing; left, upgoing.

Investigations

Hb, 13.7 g/100 ml.
WBC, 15.3×10^9/litre; predominantly neutrophils.
Sodium, 138 mmol/litre.
Potassium, 4.2 mmol/litre.
Urea, 2.3 mmol/litre.
Urinalysis, negative.

A CT scan showed oedema of the right cerebral hemisphere with obliteration of right ventricle, a right frontal collection of fluid and a markedly prominent falx.

The right frontal area was explored and 7 ml of pus removed from the subdural space; Gram's stain revealed Gram-positive cocci in chains and Gram-negative rods. She was commenced on parenteral broad-spectrum antibiotics.

Following surgery, she regained consciousness and the papilloedema resolved. However, she was left with a left hemiplegia and left homonymous hemianopia. She made steady progress until the third postoperative day when she became pyrexial, 40 °C (axilla), and developed left-sided fits.

Questions

1. What is the most likely origin of the infection?
2. Give two possible explanations for the extensive left-sided signs.
3. What two further investigations would you do at this stage?

Case 37

A 9-month-old child of non-consanguineous English parents is noted to have poor weight gain at the Well Baby Clinic. He has a good appetite and is on a mixed diet of tinned baby foods and cows' milk. Initially he was breastfed; complement milk formula feeds were introduced at 1 month and solids at 3 months. He passes one or two stools daily; they have always been bulky, loose and offensive. He had not been vomiting until recently when it had been in association with a paroxysmal cough.

The pregnancy was uncomplicated and he was born at term by spontaneous vaginal delivery; the birth weight was 3.75 kg.

He smiled at 7 weeks, rolled front to back at 6 months and sat unaided at 7 months. He now stands against the furniture · and tries to crawl.

His second triple vaccination was administered 2 weeks previously. The father is a policeman and the mother a librarian, before marriage. They live in police accommodation. There are two older normal siblings in the family.

Examination

A happy, alert child with no dysmorphic features.
Height, 71.2 cm (50th centile).
Weight, 7.87 kg (10th centile).
Pulse, 98 beats/min; sinus arrhythmia; heart sounds, normal.
Respiratory rate, 40 breaths/min; slight subcostal recession.
Breath sounds, normal.
Protuberant abdomen.
No hepatosplenomegaly.
No neurological abnormalities.

Investigations

Hb, 11.1 g/100 ml.
WBC, 6.7×10^9/litre; neutrophils, 69%; lymphocytes, 27%; monocytes, 4%.
Immunoglobulins: IgG, 6.3 g/litre (normal range, 3–12 g/litre); IgA, 0.3 g/litre (normal range, 0.2–0.8 g/litre); IgM, 0.6 g/litre (normal range, 0.2–1.0 g/litre).
Sodium, 136 mmol/litre.
Potassium, 4.2 mmol/litre.
Urea, 2.6 mmol/litre.
Blood glucose, 4.8 mmol/litre
Serum calcium, 2.3 mmol/litre.
Urinalysis, negative.
Urine culture, negative.

Chest X-ray, normal.
Bone age, 5–7 months.

Questions

1. Give three further relevant investigations.
2. Give three possible diagnoses.

Case 38

A 13-year-old girl is referred to Casualty by her general practitioner. She had been well that morning but was sent home from school complaining of headache, dizziness, difficulty in walking and finally vomiting. On questioning she said that she noticed that the letters on the blackboard had become blurred and then, later, that she staggered when she walked. The onset of symptoms had been sudden–about 3 hours prior to presentation–and had worsened rapidly. She had had one similar previous episode 9 months earlier.

She was not prone to headaches and no one in the family suffered from migraine. She had had no recent infective illnesses and no previous serious illnesses. She was happy at school, although rather shy, and was making good academic progress.

The pregnancy had been normal and she was delivered at term, needed no resuscitation and suffered no neonatal problems. Her development was normal. She was the middle child of three. Her older brother had recently left home to join the Army; she had a younger sister.

Her father suffered from trigeminal neuralgia and was treated with carbamazepine. Her mother was a well-controlled diabetic on insulin.

Examination

On examination she was apyrexial.
Height, 150 cm (10th centile).
Weight, 42 kg (25th centile).
She had breast enlargement, but had not reached her menarche.

Cardiovascular system: pulse, 120 beats/min; blood pressure, 150/110 mmHg; heart sounds, normal.

Abdominal system: low abdominal tenderness, recent perivulval bruising.

Nervous system: pupils dilated, poor response to light; fundi, disc. Margins clear.

She was unable to read the visual acuity chart.

Diplopia was demonstrated. She had an ataxic gait and poor hand and foot co-ordination.

Reflexes, brisk.

Plantars, downgoing.

Investigations

Hb, 12.1 g/100 ml.

WBC: 4.5×10^9/litre; neutrophils, 72%; lymphocytes, 24%; monocytes, 3%; eosinophils, 1%.

Sodium, 130 mmol/litre.

Potassium, 3.8 mmol/litre.

Urea, 2.6 mmol/litre

Glucose, 4.1 mmol/litre.

Plasma calcium, 2.1 mmol/litre.

Urinalysis, negative.

Lumbar puncture: lymphs, 4×10^6/litre; RBC, 200×10^6/litre; glucose, 3.0 mmol/litre; protein, 0.6 g/litre.

Skull X-ray, normal.

The symptoms remitted 4 hours after admission with no neurological sequelae.

Discussion

1. Give one further important investigation.
2. What is the most likely diagnosis?

Case 39

A 13-year-old African girl with homozygous sickle cell disease attended Outpatients complaining of rectal bleeding. Eight weeks previously she had developed a mild, diffuse abdominal discomfort followed shortly by diarrhoea, which had persisted. The stools were semi-solid and watery initially, but after 4 days she noticed occasional blood flecks. Each stool was now mixed with unaltered blood. Her bowel actions were not preceded or accompanied by an exacerbation of the abdominal discomfort or tenesmus, but for the last few days she had noted soiling on her underwear. She was unaware of being incontinent. She had lost sufficient weight to notice that her clothes were now fitting loosely.

She had not been abroad during the past year, but an uncle from Nigeria had been staying with the family for the last 4 months. No other member of the family was suffering from diarrhoea.

Sickle-cell disease had been diagnosed at 11 months of age and she had been maintained on daily folic acid supplements. She had had only a few sickle crises; her last admission had been 2 years previously.

She was one of seven children, one other of whom had sickle cell disease. Both parents were unemployed and the family lived in a damp, three-bedroomed council maisonette.

Examination

Height, 143.1 cm (3rd centile).
Weight, 28.9 kg (<3rd centile).
Conjunctivae, pale.
Pulse, 94 beats/min; blood pressure, 110/60 mm Hg.
Cardiac sounds, soft, short mid systolic murmur, maximal at left sternal edge.
Tender mass in right iliac fossa, approximately 5 × 8 cm.
No hepatosplenomegaly.

Investigations

Hb, 3 months previously 8.6 g/100 ml; now 8.3 g/100 ml.
Reticulocyte count, 7%.
Sodium, 136 mmol/litre.
Potassium, 4.1 mmol/litre.
Bicarbonate, 24 mmol/litre.
Urea, 2.7 mmol/litre.

Questions

1. Give two possible diagnoses.
2. Give two further helpful investigations to establish the diagnosis.

Case 40

A 19-month-old girl is admitted after a febrile convulsion. She had had a cough for 3 days and been pyrexial for 8 hours. Mother found her lying in a pool of vomit in bed, blue with her eyes rolled upwards.

She had been born by elective caesarean section at term, birth weight 3.57 kg. She was breastfed for 5 months, had no problems and normal developmental milestones. Over the previous winter she had had three attacks of 'wheezy bronchitis' but no previous fits. The maternal grandfather has asthma.

On examination her temperature was 41°C, she was cyanosed and twitching. Cervical lymphadenopathy was marked and respiratory rate 48 breaths/min. The throat was inflamed with no exudate and both tympanic membranes were dull. The chest was hyperinflated, breath sounds equal in right and left lungs with crepitations in the left anteriolateral area. Her pulse was 180 beats/min, her heart sounds normal. There was no hepatosplenomegaly or other positive abdominal signs and no meningism.

Investigations

Hb, 13.1 g/100 ml.
WBC: 17.8×10^9/litre; neutrophils, 79%; lymphocytes, 20%.
Platelets, normal.
CSF: micros, 30×10^3/cmm RBC, no WBC; culture, no growth.
Blood culture, no growth.
Throat swab, no growth.
Mantoux test, negative.
Chest X-ray, linear shadowing, left mid-zone.
    She was treated with ampicillin and flucloxacillin intravenously,

but on changing to oral antibiotics 2 days later she became irritable and pyrexial. Repeat lumbar puncture was traumatic.
CSF: micros, RBC, 2378×10^6/litre; WBC, 91×10^6/litre; lymphs, 28×10^6/litre.
Gram's stain, no organisms seen.
    Chloramphenicol was added to the medication. The temperature settled and her general condition improved.
    Three days later she was noted to have markedly decreased chest movements on the left, the percussion note was hyper-resonant on the left and breath sounds were reduced. The following day a 'brassy cough' developed; chest signs were unchanged. Repeat chest X-ray showed hyperinflation of the left lung.

Questions

1. What is the diagnosis?
2. What is the treatment?

Case 41

A 10-year-old boy is referred to Outpatients from a country residential home with a provisional diagnosis of retinoblastoma. He had complained of poor vision in the right eye and was noted to have absence of the red reflex and a white raised plaque arising from the temporal side of the retina. No systemic abnormalities were noted.
    In Outpatients the boy complained of no symptoms other than of visual loss. His housemother stated that he was generally healthy, had a good appetite and did not become unduly tired on physical exertion. He was of average intelligence with an IQ of 90. No pets were allowed in the Children's Home.
    He had been taken into care 2 years previously following the prosecution of his parents for child abuse, at which time a small white fibrotic lesion was noted in the temporal area of the right retina during his admission examination. He was the third of five children; two others were also in care. The family had lived in a terraced house which faced an area of wasteland on which the children played.

Examination

Height, 142 cm (75th centile).
Weight, 31 kg (75th centile).
Apyrexial, no skin rashes.
Cardiovascular and respiratory systems normal; no hepatosplenomegaly; no abdominal masses. Small, firm inguinal lymph nodes were palpable bilaterally.
Pupils equal and reacting to light, no proptosis.
Fundi, left, normal; right, large white raised irregular plaque.
Visual fields, large scotoma in right nasal field.
Reflexes, normal.
Plantars, downgoing.

Investigations

Hb, 12.5 mg/100 ml.
WBC, 16.7×10^9/litre; neutrophils, 43%; lymphocytes, 10%; eosinophils, 35%; monocytes, 3%.
Skull and chest X-ray, normal.
Urinalysis, normal.

Questions

1. Give one further important investigation.
2. What is the most likely diagnosis?

Case 42

An 18-month-old boy was admitted from the Middle East with bone disease. He had been a full-term, normal delivery weighing approximately 3 kg. He appeared normal at birth but had failed to thrive since. On admission he weighed 6.8 kg, height was 70 cm (well below 3rd centile) and head circumference on the 50th centile. He had had constipation for some weeks and vomiting for the last 3 days.

Developmental milestones were not known, but he had never

been able to walk. His mother was aged 35 and father aged 48; they were first cousins. Six siblings aged 12–17 were alive and well, but four others had all died of 'vomiting' aged less than 1 year.

On examination he was an extremely wasted child, dehydrated with gross rickets. Respiratory rate was 40 beats/min but the chest was clear and heart sounds normal.

The abdomen was generally distended, liver edge just palpable, bowel sounds absent, and rectal examination revealed hard, formed stool.

In the CNS he was markedly apathetic and lethargic with reduced tone but no focal signs.

Investigations

Hb, 13.3 g/100 ml.
WBC: 12.0×10^9/litre; neutrophils, 71% with left shift.
Urea, 7.2 mmol/litre.
Sodium, 126 mmol/litre.
Potassium, 1.4 mmol/litre.
Bicarbonate, 11 mmol/litre.
Blood sugar, 3.5 mmol/litre.
Phosphate, 0.94 mmol/litre.
Calcium, 2.1 mmol/litre.
Alkaline phosphatase, 1560 iu/litre.
Chest X-ray: lung fields clear; heart normal. Extensive loss of bone trabeculae in the ribs and a number of fractures present.
Limb X-rays: gross demineralization of all bones. Appearance consistent with rickets, possibly associated with vitamin D deficiency.
Urine analysis, pH 6.0; protein, +; glucose, trace.

Questions

1. What is the diagnosis?
2. What is the most likely cause?
3. What three further investigations would you do to confirm the diagnosis?
4. What are the three most important factors in long-term management of this child?
5. Name two other causes of this syndrome.

Case 43

A 14-year-old boy was referred to a child guidance clinic for assessment of episodes of uncontrollable aggression. He had been an affectionate and placid child until he was 8 years old when his parents separated and his father refused to see the children. He gradually became withdrawn and had aggressive outbursts when confronted by his mother over any misdemeanour. However, over the past 13 months some episodes had become unpredictable and were usually associated with abdominal pain. The general practitioner initially diagnosed abdominal migraine and prescribed analgesics and laxatives but to no effect; it was then suggested that the diagnosis was temporal lobe epilepsy. An EEG was normal and a trial of carbamazepine failed to relieve the attacks. The child was then referred to child guidance. He was seen at the initial interview with his mother and 11-year-old sister; it was felt that individual psychotherapy was appropriate.

The father was a lock-keeper and the family had lived in a cottage by the lock. Father and son had spent a great deal of time together, either on their own boat or fishing. However, the father was made redundant and the family had to move to the local town, where the mother gained employment as a domestic cleaning lady. Thereafter the relationship between husband and wife deteriorated and he eventually left. The child interpreted this as the mother forcing the father to go because he did not have a job, and refusing access to the children. He, therefore, reacted aggressively towards correction and expressed a desire to kill his mother. He was frank about these emotions but was puzzled about, and scared of, his unpredictable outbursts.

During one such aggressive episode he became violent and the police were called. They took him to the local police station where he was seen by a police surgeon and referred to the Accident and Emergency Department.

Examination

Aggressive, unco-operative child.
Height, 163.9 cm (75th centile).
Weight, 48.9 kg (50th centile).
Pyrexial, 38.4 °C.

No clinical jaundice or anaemia.
Pulse, 112 beats/min; blood pressure, 140/90 mmHg.
Soft, mid systolic murmur in the pulmonary area varied with position.
No hepatosplenomegaly.
Left otitis media.
Neurological system–refused to answer questions. Pupils, reacted to light.
Fundi, normal.
Loss of deep tendon reflexes; plantars, downgoing.
Pigmented areas on forearms, back of hands and malar region of the face. Evidence of secondary sexual development: enlargement of penis and testes, scanty pubic hair; his voice had broken.

Investigations

Hb, 14.1 g/100 ml.
WBC, 15.6×10^9/litre.
Sodium, 128 mmol/litre.
Potassium, 4.6 mmol/litre.
Glucose, 6.7 mmol/litre.
Urea, 7.4 mmol/litre.

Questions

1. What is the most likely diagnosis?
2. What is the inheritance of the disease?

Case 44

An 11-week-old male infant was brought to Casualty with a history of lethargy, poor feeding and weight loss. He was a full-term baby, normal delivery, birth weight 3.1 kg, and had had no perinatal problems. He had been seen in Casualty 4 weeks previously with vomiting and had been treated with clear fluids. A follow-up outpatient appointment was made but he never attended. Apparently he had gradually become less interested in his feeds, eventually taking approximately 2 fluid oz (57 ml) per feed three to four times a day. There had been occasional vomits but no diarrhoea. Various milks had been tried, with little success.

The parents were not married. His mother was English, aged 22 years, and had married a Thai man in order for him to gain entry to the UK. She was co-habiting with another Thai man, the father of the child, who was due to return to Thailand in the near future.

On examination the baby was marasmic, weighing 2.9 kg. He was miserable with an anxious look and ammoniacal nappy rash, but no other abnormality. He was admitted to hospital and given regular feeds of a normal formula baby milk at 150 ml/kg daily. Initially he took feeds eagerly and gained weight, but after 2 days became uninterested. Tube feeding resulted in a marked increase in vomiting but no diarrhoea.

Investigations

Hb, 11.4 g/100 ml.
WBC: 14.2×10^9/litre–normal differential; film, normal.
Urea, 2.0 mmol/litre.
Sodium, 137 mmol/litre.
Potassium, 3.8 mmol/litre.
Chloride, 100 mmol/l.
Bicarbonate, 30 mmol/litre.
Urine microscopy and culture, normal.
Stool culture, no pathogens.
Urine: reducing substances, negative; 24-hour VMA excretion, normal.
Chest X-ray, normal.

Questions

1. Give three possible diagnoses in order of priority.
2. Give three investigations that you would carry out immediately to help prove the most likely diagnosis.

Case 45

A 15-year-old primigravida schoolgirl was admitted in established labour. The pregnancy had been concealed until late and she had not attended any antenatal clinics. Her periods had been irregular before pregnancy, but the head was engaged and the fundal height was compatible with a term pregnancy. Labour proceeded uneventfully and she was delivered of a normal female infant. Apgar scores were 7 at 1 min and 9 at 5 min. Birth weight, 3.51 kg. Breastfeeding was attempted unsuccessfully and bottle feeding was commenced on day 4. On day 3 the baby was noticed to be jaundiced, serum bilirubin 186 μmol/litre; this rose to 225 μmol/litre the following day and she was treated effectively with intermittent phototherapy for 3 days. However, the jaundice recurred after the cessation of treatment and it was noticed that there had been poor weight gain. She had lost 196 g in the first 2 days and subsequently had gained only 15 g. Phototherapy was recommenced and she had supplementary feeds via an indwelling nasogastric tube. On day 10 she was still jaundiced and had now developed non-bloody diarrhoea and vomiting.

Examination

Weight, 3.415 kg.
Clinically jaundiced.
Pulse, 138 beats/min; blood pressure, 65/40 mmHg.
Heart sounds, normal.
Hepar, 3.5 cm.
No splenomegaly.
Lethargic but irritable on handling.
Tone, poor.

Investigations

Hb, 14.7 g/100 ml.
WBC, 11.6 $\times$ 10^9/litre.
Glucose, 1.9 mmol/litre.
Bilirubin, 186 μmol/litre.
PTT/KCT, prolonged.
Blood gases: pH, 7.29; $P\text{co}_2$, 4.2 KPa; $P\text{o}_2$, 11.7 KPa; bicarbonate,

21.3 mmol; base excess, 6.7 mmol/litre; standard bicarbonate, 18 mmol/litre; standard base excess, 7.0 mmol/litre. Lumbar puncture: lymphocyte 3×10^6/litre; protein, 0.4 g/litre; glucose, 1.6 mmol/litre.

Antibodies to: toxoplasma, 1:8; cytomegalovirus, 1:8; rubella, 1:16; herpes, 1:8.

Urinalysis, Clinitest positive.

Stool-reducing substances, negative.

Questions

1. Give two possible diagnoses.
2. Give three further important investigations.

Case 46

A 10-year-old boy who has completed $2\frac{1}{2}$ years of treatment for common acute lymphoblastic leukaemia (ALL) on a United Kingdom Acute Lymphoblastic Leukaemia (trial) (UKALL) regimen without relapse and been off treatment for 7 months presents with a mild pyrexia and generalized pains. Three weeks previously he had had a heavy cold along with the rest of his family and following this he had gradually developed swelling of his ankles and elbows. Five days before he had been reluctant to go to school in the morning, walked slowly and refused to put on his coat despite the cold weather. After 2 days of similar behaviour his mother realized that he could not extend his elbows. He had lost 4 kg in weight even though his appetite was fair.

His father worked as a dental technician and mother as a barmaid. There was a brother aged 16 years. All were in good health.

Examination

Height, 136.5 cm (50th centile).
Weight, 26.5 kg (25th centile).
Pyrexial, 37.8 °C (oral).
Pulse, 97 beats/min; sinus arrhythmia.

Blood pressure, 110/70 mmHg.
Heart sounds, normal.
Chest, clear.
Abdomen, normal.
Mouth, no discoloration.
Tongue, marginal atrophy.
Cranial nerves, unable to protrude tongue fully.
Erythematous rash on upper eyelids, shoulders, upper chest and front of thighs.
Non-pitting oedema of both feet and ankles to mid-calf level and around elbows. Generalized muscle wasting with fasciculation, marked over upper limb girdle.
Movement in all joints painful.
Neck: limited extension, rotation; flexion normal.
Elbows, 110° fixed flexion.
Shoulders, 90° abduction.
Fingers, difficulty with fine movements.
Hips, flexion 45°.
Ankles, painless normal movement.

Investigations

Hb, 13.7 g/100 ml.
ESR, 4 mm in first hour.
WBC: 12.5 × 10^9/litre; neutrophils, 80%; lymphocytes, 12%; monocytes, 8%.
Platelets, 251 × 10^9/litre,
Urea, 6.1 mmol/litre.
Calcium, 2.25 mmol/litre.
Sodium, 136 mmol/litre.
Potassium, 4.2 mmol/litre.
Total protein, 66 g/litre.
Alkaline phosphatase, 319 iu.
X-rays, elbow and ankles, NAD.
Chest X-ray, no abnormality.
Immunoglobulins: IgG, IgA, IgM, normal.
Urinalysis, NAD.

Questions

1. What are two differential diagnoses?
2. What three investigations would you do immediately?

3. What three other physical signs might one expect to see or develop?

Case 47

An 8-year-old girl is referred to Outpatients with a 4-month history of headaches and vomiting. She had been treated by her general practitioner with analgesics and antiemetics but these had afforded only temporary relief.

The headaches were frontal, not throbbing and were usually present on awakening but tended to improve during the day. The vomiting was variable but was not associated with any foodstuffs or accompanied by nausea. These episodes occurred on any day and did not resolve at the weekends or during school holidays. There was no aura and she was not drowsy or disorientated either during or after the episode. She had never suffered a convulsion and there was no family history of fits.

The pregnancy had been normal and there were no problems in the neonatal or infantile periods. She sat at 6 months, walked at 14 months and was reported as average in school.

The family lived in an old terraced house in an industrial area. The house had recently been replumbed and redecorated. Her father was a 46-year-old steel worker and her mother, aged 39 years, worked part-time in a factory canteen. There were three healthy siblings aged 12, 9 and 5 years.

Examination

Height, 126.4 cm (75th centile).
Weight, 28.7 kg (90th centile).
Apyrexial.
Pulse, 68 beats/min; sinus arrhythmia; blood pressure, 125/85 mmHg.
Peripheral pulses, normal.
No added heart sounds.
ENT: healthy tympanic membranes, positive light reflexes.
No abdominal masses.
Pupils, equal and reacting to light.

Fundi, discs pink, veins engorged.
No nystagmus.
Cranial nerves, no abnormality.
Power, normal in all limbs.
Gait, unsteady, wide based.
Standing and sitting, truncal ataxia.
Co-ordination, upper limbs good; lower limbs, poor.
Heel–shin test, normal; sensation, normal.
Reflexes: normal plantars, extensor.

Investigations

Hb, 14.1 g/100 ml.
WBC, 6.8 × 10^9/litre.
Sodium, 139 mmol/litre.
Potassium, 4.3 mmol/litre.
Urea, 2.1 mmol/litre
Protoporphyrins 24 ng/dl (normal range < 50 ng/dl).
ECG axis, +85°.
Skull X-ray: erosion of the posterior clinoid process.

Questions

1. What is the most likely diagnosis?
2. Give one further important investigation.

Case 48

An 8-year-old boy with Down's syndrome was admitted for revision of the distal catheter of his atrioventricular Spitz–Holter valve. The valve had been inserted at 10 weeks of age and had required revision once only at 3 years of age.

He was born at 39 weeks' gestation by dates, birth weight 2.37 kg, to a 42-year-old mother after a normal pregnancy. The diagnosis of trisomy 21 was made clinically at birth and confirmed on chromosome analysis. On the second day of life he developed mild jaundice and a diffuse but discrete, erythe-matous maculopapular rash. The rash cleared within the first week, the jaundice within the first 3 weeks.

Both parents rejected him initially but, after counselling, they accepted him home aged 17 days.

He was seen regularly in Outpatients where it was noticed that his head circumference was increasing rapidly. CT scan at 10 weeks had demonstrated dilated lateral ventricles and an atrio-ventricular valve was inserted.

He was able to walk unaided but was unable to help in dressing or undressing. He was unable to talk but would obey simple commands. He attended a school for the severely educa-tionally subnormal.

He was the third child; the other siblings were 18 and 20 years old and both had left home. The family now lived in a two-bedroomed flat over their fish and chip shop.

Examination

Height, 113.3 cm (3rd centile).
Weight, 21.7 kg (10th centile).
Many stigmata of trisomy 21.
Pulse, 98 beats/min.
Heart sounds: apex, short mid systolic murmur, long diastolic murmur; base, ejection systolic murmur.
Breath sounds, normal.
No hepatosplenomegaly.
Responded to simple commands, e.g. shut the door.
Pupils, equal and reactive to light; no cataracts.
Fundi, bilateral diffuse choroidoretinitis.
Reflexes, normal.
Plantars, downgoing.

Investigation

ECG: sinus rhythm, left axis deviation.

Questions

1. Give one further important investigation.
2. Give two possible diagnoses.

Case 49

A $7\frac{1}{2}$-year-old boy is referred to Outpatients for investigation of recurrent abdominal pain over the last 18 months. The attacks occurred at 4-monthly intervals initially, but more recently every 4–6 weeks, on occasion necessitating sending the boy home from school. His general practitioner had never found any positive physical signs but treated him for a possible urinary tract infection with antibiotics. The episodes of pain would start on the left side of the abdomen, any time of the day or night, and gradually become generalized. At the same time he became pyrexial, his temperature ranging up to 39 °C; he was flushed, agitated and nauseated with copious vomiting but no diarrhoea. There were no urinary symptoms. At these times he liked to go to bed and after approximately 24 hours the pain would suddenly resolve and within 1 hour he would be back to his normal self.

He was a full-term normal delivery with no problems apart from being a 'sickly' baby. He is the only natural child of the parents, who are both English. His mother is a registered childminder. Another boy, 16 months younger, with asthma and eczema, has been living with the family for about 3 years on long-term fostering. The father works as a head porter in a block of flats. Family relationships are said to be good and school work satisfactory.

On examination there were no abnormal physical signs.

Investigations

Full blood count (FBC), normal.
ESR, 3 mm in first hour.
MSU: micros, less than 3×10^9 WBC/litre; culture, no significant growth.
Urinalysis, negative.
Urine porphobilinogen, normal.

Questions

1. What two further points in the history would you like to know?
2. What two steps would you take to help you make a diagnosis?

Case 50

An 8-year-old boy is admitted via Casualty for the third time in 3 months with similar symptoms of severe pain at the tip of the penis on micturition, frequency and lower abdominal pain. He had been enuretic all his life. He had first developed these symptoms 17 months earlier. Nothing was found on examination and investigation showed no urinary tract infection and a normal IVP. He improved spontaneously but had a similar episode lasting 5 weeks, 6 months later.

He was admitted for investigation 14 months after the initial episode. Expression cystogram done under general anaesthetic was normal, and he was left catheterized for 24 hours because of difficulty in passing the cystoscope. On catheter removal he continued to have severe difficulty in passing urine and required another general anaesthetic for insertion of a suprapubic catheter.

He gradually improved. Erythromycin was given for treatment of urethritis but no cause was found. Two weeks after admission he developed vomiting and upper abdominal pain; there was nothing to find on examination and he was discharged home 5 days later, still vomiting occasionally.

He was re-admitted 1 week later and had another general anaesthetic for cystourethroscopy. Urethral stricture was found with a proximally dilatated urethra and a hypertrophied bladder. A suprapubic catheter was inserted and erythromycin re-started. Two further urethral dilatations were done during the next 10 days, both under general anaesthetic. Prior to the second, 'odd' behaviour was noted, in that he was screaming inappropriately, soiling deliberately and biting the thermometer. He continued to be 'difficult' on the ward and 1 week later, when ready to go home, he started vomiting, screaming and complaining of substernal pain and headache. Mother did not want her son to have psychiatric help and he was discharged still on erythromycin.

On his third admission, 5 weeks later, he developed acute urinary retention. Expression cystogram under general anaesthetic revealed a markedly dilated urethra except for the final 1 cm which was severely constricted. An extensive meatotomy was done and suprapubic catheter inserted. Nausea, vomiting, abdominal pain and mild drowsiness developed 5 days after the operation.

Examination

Height, 126.5 cm (50th centile).
Weight, 21.0 kg (10th centile).
Pyrexial, 37.4 °C (oral).
Fully conscious and orientated.
Mild jaundice.
Pulse, 90 beats/min, regular; blood pressure, 100/70 mmHg.
Heart sounds, normal.
Chest, clear.
Fauces, normal.
No lymphadenopathy.
Abdomen: liver, tipped, non-tender; spleen, not palpable; no ascites.
No tremor or flap.
No focal neurological signs.

Investigations

Hb, 11.8 g/100 ml.
WBC: 10.6×10^9/litre; neutrophils, 54%; lymphocytes, 38%; eosinophils, 1%; monocytes, 8%.
Film: target cells, some active lymphocytes.
Platelets, 218×10^9/litre.
Monospot, negative.
Prothrombin time, 59 s; control, 14 s.
Activated partial thrombopastin time (APTT) 98 s; control, 35 s.

Table 1 Initial results (normal range) and results taken 2 weeks later

Test	Initial results	Results 2 weeks later
Total bilirubin (mmol/litre)	80	480
Conjugated bilirubin (mmol/litre)	40	270
Alkaline phosphatase (iu/litre)	685	995
ALT (iu/litre)	1379	170
AST (iu/litre)	1110	385
Albumin (g/litre)	33	26
IgG (g/litre)	7.5 (5–14)	12.7
IgA (g/litre)	1.7 (0.5–2.5)	2.2
IgM (g/litre)	8.0 (0.5–2.0)	3.1

Anti-hepatitis A virus IgM, negative.
Hepatitis B surface antigen, negative.
Cytomegalovirus (CMV) IgM, negative.
Epstein–Barr virus (EBV) IgM, negative.
Herpes simplex IgM, negative.
MSU, NAD.
Stools: no ova or cysts; no pathogens grown.
Autoantibodies: smooth muscle, 1+; liver–kidney microsomes, strongly positive; all others, negative.
Ammonia, 139 μmol/litre (normal < 40).

Questions

1. What three differential diagnoses would you consider most likely?
2. What four important investigations would you do?
3. What three necessary steps in treatment would you start?

Case 51

A 3-year-old child attended Outpatients for cyanotic episodes. The first episode had been 7 months previously. The child had had an upper respiratory tract infection and on going to sleep she began to snore and then became cyanosed. The episode was aborted when the mother awoke the child and sat her upright. The next episode was several weeks later. The episode again occurred as the child was going to sleep and aborted as before. The attacks became more frequent, especially if associated with an upper respiratory tract infection, all occurring on falling asleep and all easily aborted. The child had never developed stridor, had had no cyanotic episodes whilst awake, but was a mouth-breather.

She was a term infant, born vaginally, birth weight 3.24 kg. She was the third child. The father, aged 41 years, was a miner and the mother, aged 36 years, was a food packer at the local factory. The family lived in a two-bedroomed terraced house with open-coal fires.

Examination

Apyrexial.
Height, 90.7 cm (25th centile).
Weight, 13.2 kg (25th centile).
Pulse, 90 beats/min; blood pressure, 80/55 mmHg.
Parasternal heave.
Apex beat, mid clavicular line, fifth interspace; second sound wide-splitting–moving with respiration.
No murmurs.
Peripheral pulses, normal.
Mouth-breathing.
No added respiratory sounds.
No abdominal or neurological abnormalities.

Investigations

Hb, 12.1 g/100 ml.
WBC, 5.9×10^9/litre.
Chest X-ray–enlarged cardiac shadow.
ECG: axis +90°; right ventricular hypertrophy.

Table 1 Cardiac catheter studies

Pressures (mmHg)	Oxygen saturation (%)
Superior vena cava	69
Right atrium, m = 6	67
Right ventricle 110/6	66
Pulmonary artery 105/45	66
Pulmonary wedge pressure 5	

Questions

1. What is the most likely aetiology of her cardiovascular problems?

Case 52

A 7-year-old girl presents with a 3-month history of pain in the shoulders, elbows, hips and knees. Her parents feel that she is not as active as she used to be; in particular she has not been able to walk as far as before, one of the family's favourite pursuits being hiking. At the end of the day she feels weak but is not anxious to go upstairs to bed. Apart from this her general health has been good with no intercurrent infections and no previous history of note. She has a brother and sister, both of whom are older and who are well. There has been no recent illness in the family.

She was seen by her general practitioner, who could find no abnormal clinical signs and prescribed aspirin. The pain improved but she appeared to get weaker.

On examination she was apyrexial with no rash or lymphadenopathy. General examination of heart, chest and abdomen and central nervous system was normal apart from slightly reduced tendon reflexes.

Musculoskeletal examination revealed no abnormality in the joints and non-tender muscles. The facial expression was normal but neck extension and shoulder adduction were weak, and there was slight winging of both scapulae. She had a waddling gait, difficulty in getting off the floor without assistance and weakness of the gluteal muscles. Other muscles appeared normal.

Investigations

Hb, 12 g/100 ml.
WBC: 6.3 × 10^9/litre; neutrophils, 46%; lymphocytes, 49%; eosinophils, 3%; basophils, 2%.
Platelets, 320 × 10^9/litre.
Paul–Bunnell test, negative.
ESR, 15 mm in first hour.
AST, normal.
ALT, normal.
Alkaline phosphatase, 320 units.
Antistreptolysin O titre (ASOT), <60 units.
Antinuclear antibody (ANA), negative.
Rheumatoid factor (RF), negative.
Throat swab: β-haemolytic streptococci, group B.
Nose swab, Staphylococcus aureus.

Questions

1. What is the most likely diagnosis?
2. What three investigations would you carry out to aid diagnosis?

Case 53

A 14-year-old boy was admitted with a chest infection and right-sided heart failure. He suffered from chronic granulomatous disease and had had recurrent chest infections. These had produced sufficient lung damage to cause incipient cor pulmonale. He was maintained on regular digoxin and also salbutamol, which improved his peak flow.

He had had a bone marrow transplant 3 years previously from a related donor. The graft had taken initially but then gradually failed as his own marrow regenerated. No further transplants had been attempted.

He had developed a cough 4 days prior to this admission. He had been commenced on co-trimoxazole immediately, but he had gradually worsened and was admitted with a productive cough and right-sided failure.

He had been adopted at the age of 5 years. His adoptive parents, who had one son of their own, had been fully conversant with his condition at the time of adoption.

He attended the local comprehensive school, but had additional private tuition to minimize the effect of repeated hospital admissions.

Examination

Height, 140.2 cm (< 3rd centile).
Weight, 32.7 kg (< 3rd centile).
Centrally cyanosed.
Pulse, 112 beats/min; blood pressure, 110/70 mmHg.
Parasternal heave.
Mid systolic ejection murmur, maximal in the pulmonary area.
Hyperinflated chest with increased anteroposterior diameter–poor respiratory excursion–accessory respiratory muscles used.

Bilateral scattered crepitations and rhonchi.
Smooth, non-tender hepatomegaly of 2 cm.
Deformity of left upper arm and right femur from episodes of osteomyelitis.

Investigations

Hb, 14.6 g/100 ml.
WBC: 15.7 × 10^9/litre; neutrophils, 73%; lymphocytes, 24%; monocytes, 2%; eosinophils., 1%. pH 7.36.
Po_2, 7.5 kPa.
Pco_2, 6.9 kPa.
Bicarbonate, 31 mmol/litre.
Base excess, 5 mmol/litre.
   He was given oxygen by mask and commenced on carbenicillin and tobramycin. Theophylline was added in view of worsened wheezing. He improved gradually and after 48 hours was no longer cyanosed; however, he was noted to have coupling beats.

Questions

1. What are the two most important investigations?

Case 54

A 14-month-old Bangladeshi boy was referred with a 1-month history of 'eye problems'. The father was a very poor historian, and mother spoke no English. The eyes were said to be flitting from side to side. His appetite had decreased over the previous 6 months but there were no other symptoms of note.
   He had been a full-term, normal delivery weighing 2.46 kg with no neonatal problems, the first child of unrelated parents. He was breastfed for 8 months, then his mother had become pregnant again, so he was weaned on to a proprietary milk, together with some solid food such as rice. He had occasional vomits but no

diarrhoea. His weight had been on the 25th centile until the age of 9 months, but since then had gradually fallen on to the 3rd centile. His height had always been on the 25th centile. Head circumference, 47 cm (50th centile). Milestones were normal and immunizations given in full .

His father was unemployed and the family had lived with paternal grandparents in council accommodation until recently when they had been asked to leave. Since then they had lived in a squat with very poor facilities.

On examination he was an active, thin but very happy child. No abnormality could be found except for gross nystagmus present in all directions. He was seen by an ophthalmologist who thought the fundi looked normal and diagnosed congenital nystagmus of unknown aetiology.

Following admission to hospital he remained a poor feeder. His mother was encouraged to feed him frequently. She had already delivered at 7 months, the baby being in another hospital. Tube feeding was started because of poor weight gain, with a small degree of success. Extra calories were added to a milk-based feed. Since the parents were agitating to go home, the tube was removed and frequent feeds given by the nurses. Despite adequate calorie intake, the weight remained static. On discharge of the premature baby, the parents insisted on having both children at home. Following discharge he started to lose weight again; the parents had not made up feeds as instructed, and were not feeding him on a regular basis. Despite his emaciation he remained an active, happy child.

Investigations

Hb, 12.2 g/100 ml.
WBC: 13.9 × 10^9/litre, film, normal.
Urea, 3.7 mmol/litre.
Sodium, 139 mmol/litre.
Potassium, 4.2 mmol/litre.
Bicarbonate, 21 mmol/litre.
Venous pH, 7.42.
Alkaline phosphatase, 418 iu/litre.
ALT, 8 iu/litre.
AST, 20 iu/litre.
Calcium, 2.30 mmol/litre.

Phosphate, 1.5 mmol/litre.
Total protein, 60 g/litre.
Albumin, 34 g/litre.
Chest X-ray, normal.
Bone age, just over 1 year.
MSU, NAD.
Stool: semi-solid specimen; micros, no ova or parasites seen; culture, enteropathogenic *Escherichia coli* 026 isolated.
Xylose level, 1 hour absorption test, 2.28 mmol/litre.
Sweat sodium, 15 mmol/litre.
Sweat chloride, 4 mmol/litre.
Urinalysis, NAD.

Questions

1. What two further investigations are required?
2. What is the most likely diagnosis?
3. What is the treatment?

Case 55

A 4-year-old boy is brought to Casualty. He arrived in England 4 days previously, having lived in Turkey for the majority of his life. Two days ago he had developed a mild fever associated with a cough and headache. Central abdominal pain, apparently dull and constant, had been present for 24 hours and his appetite was poor.

He had been born by normal delivery but the length of gestation was uncertain. He was breastfed for 6 months and his weight gain was good. At 9 months he developed a chest infection, and at 2 years had severe gastroenteritis following which he had made slow weight gain for some months. Developmental milestones were within normal limits.

The father works in the Turkish Consulate and the mother is a housewife; both are well. There is one 18-month-old female sibling who had gastroenteritis 2 months previously but is now well.

Examination

Mild pallor.
Throat slightly inflamed.
Cervical lymphadenopathy, nodes small and non-tender.
Tympanic membranes, positive light reflexes.
Chest clear.
Pulse 90 beats/min, regular; blood pressure 90/60 mm Hg.
Heart sounds normal.
Abdomen slightly distended, mild generalized tenderness, bowel sounds present.
Liver 1 cm below the costal margin; no spleen palpable.
Minimal meningism.

Initial investigations

Hb, 9.0 g/100 ml.
WBC: 4.0×10^9/litre; neutrophils, 25%; lymphocytes, 62%; eosinophils, 5%; monocytes, 6%; basophils, 2%.
Platelets, 203×10^9/litre.
Throat swab, no growth.
CSF: not under pressure; micros, no cells seen; culture, no growth.
Chest X-ray, clear.
Bilirubin, 34 mmol/litre.
Alkaline phosphatase, 490 iu/litre.
AST, 25 iu/litre.
ALT, 20 iu/litre.
Urinalysis, NAD.
   He is admitted for observation but promptly starts vomiting and the temperature continues on an upward trend. On and off he appears disorientated and on the fourth day after admission he has a generalized convulsion lasting approximately 1 min. On examination immediately afterwards he is a little drowsy and physical signs appear unchanged. Meningism is difficult to assess, but is not obviously present and the fundi are normal.

Further investigations

Hb, 7 g/100 ml.
WBC: 3.2×10^9/litre; neutrophils, 22%; lymphocytes, 60%.

Platelets, 250×10^9/litre.
CSF: traumatic tap; RBC, 18×10^6/litre; WBC, 18 neutrophils; 30 lymphocytes $\times 10^6$/litre; sugar, 3.3 mmol/litre.
Blood sugar, 4.2 mmol/litre.
Calcium, 2.1 mmol/litre.
Urea, 7.5 mmol/litre.
Sodium, 134 mmol/litre.
Potassium, 3.2 mmol/litre.
Occult test on stools, strongly positive.

Questions

1. What is the most likely diagnosis?
2. Give two investigations.
3. What is the treatment of choice?

Case 56

A 3-year-old boy presents to his general practitioner with pain and a slight limp of his left leg. A week earlier he had had 'flu', consisting of a mild fever, coryza and being generally 'off colour'. Initially he had appeared to improve, but 2 days previously he had become febrile again with headache and irritability. He complained of pain in the left leg and back the next day, and when he started limping his parents became concerned.

The family were living on a gypsy encampment in a caravan. The camp population was very mobile with many stray animals around. Many of the amenities had been smashed so that lavatories and washrooms provided unsatisfactory sanitation. The father worked in the 'car trade' and the mother was unemployed and illiterate. There were six other children ranging from 4 to 18 years. School attendance had been sporadic. General health was good, but both the grandfather who lived with the family and mother had been treated for tuberculosis some 5 years ago. A couple of children on the camp had also had 'flu'. In the past the patient had been born 'at home', bottlefed and had only been seen twice by a doctor for scabies and tonsillitis.

Examination

Miserable but co-operative child.
Height, 98.7 cm (90th centile).
Weight, 15.6 kg (75th centile).
Pyrexial, 38.2 °C (axilla).
Pulse, 110/min; sinus arrhythmia; blood pressure, 100/60 mmHg.
Heart sounds, normal.
Chest, clear.
Fauces, mildly inflamed.
Tympanic membranes, normal.
Non-tender tonsillar lymphadenopathy.
Abdomen, normal.
Mild nuchal rigidity.
Pupils equal, reacted to light; fundi, normal.
Cranial nerves, normal.
Left foot drop.
Decreased tone, left leg.
Absent left ankle reflex and plantar response.
Tender right thigh.
Sensation normal.

Investigations

Hb, 12.6 g/100 ml.
WBC: 8.3×10^9/litre; neutrophils, 42%; lymphocytes, 55%; eosinophils, 3%.
Platelets, 204×10^9/litre.
Chest X-ray, normal. X-ray, hips and leg, normal.
Urea, 4.1 mmol/litre.
Electrolytes, normal.
Blood sugar, 4.2 mmol/litre.
Calcium, 2.1 mmol/litre.
Throat swab, no growth.

Questions

1. What is the diagnosis?
2. What two investigations would you do?
3. What three important steps would you undertake in management?

Case 57

A 29-year-old primigravida was admitted at approximately 36 weeks' gestation in early labour. She was experiencing uterine contractions every 10 min and had been doing so for the 90 min prior to admission. On vaginal examination the os cervix was still closed.

She had attended antenatal clinics regularly after booking in at 12 weeks' gestation. She was 1.5 m tall and weighed 42.2 kg at booking. Weight gain had been satisfactory, blood pressure stable and routine haematology and serology normal throughout the pregnancy.

Two hours after admission she began to vomit. She was apyrexial and no abnormality was found on examination. Microscopy of urine revealed no WBC or micro-organisms and a peripheral blood film did not show a leukocytosis. An intravenous infusion of 5% dextrose was commenced at 250 ml/hour and she was given 12.5 mg prochlorperazine as an intramuscular injection. The vomiting persisted for a further 3 hours and then ceased. The intravenous infusion of 5% dextrose was continued at 250 ml/hour for a further 3 hours, then reduced to 150 ml/hour until delivery 13 hours later despite an infusion of oxytocin.

She was delivered of a normal male infant who required no resuscitation, birth weight 2.12 kg. Mother and child were transferred to the postnatal ward. At the age of 3 hours the infant had a generalized convulsion lasting 1–2 min and he was transferred to a special care baby unit where an immediate Dextrostix registered 4–6 mmol/litre.

Examination demonstrated no abnormal or dysmorphic features and he was apyrexial.

Investigations

Hb, 17.3 g/100 ml.
WBC, 14.2×10^9/litre.
Blood sugar, 7.4 mmol/litre.
pH, 7.37.
P_{O_2}, 10.7 kPa.
P_{CO_2}, 5.6 kPa.
Bicarbonate, 21 mmol/litre.
Base excess, 4 mmol/litre.

Lumbar puncture: RBC, 4×10^6/litre; lymphs, 2×10^6/litre, no organisms seen.

Serum was taken for viral titres.

Bacterial swabs taken from ear, throat, nose, rectum and mother's vagina.

The infant continued fitting intermittently. The convulsions were generalized and short-lasting—less than 1–2 min. Intravenous diazepam 0.5 mg did not control the fitting.

Questions

1. What is the most likely cause of this baby's fits?
2. Give one vital investigation.

Case 58

A 5-month-old male infant is admitted with diarrhoea and vomiting associated with failure to thrive. He was the third child of an Irish family with two healthy female sibs aged 2 and 5. The family lived in a two-bedroomed council flat on social security.

Birth history was normal, birth weight 3.5 kg. He had no neonatal problems and was bottlefed. He was first admitted at the age of 2 months with loose stools and poor weight gain; weight was 4.2 kg. He was given clear fluids and then regraded on to his usual bottle milk. He gradually gained weight in hospital and was discharged after 10 days. At home he failed to gain any more weight and was re-admitted 4 weeks later. A low-lactose milk was substituted and he again started to gain weight. Following discharge he was initially well and cereals were introduced. However, he required further admission with vomiting, loose stools and respiratory tract infection at 4 months. He improved with antibiotics. In view of his continuing poor weight he had the following investigations:

Barium meal and follow-through, normal.

Sweat test: sodium, 35 mmol/litre.

Jejunal biopsy, minimal villous atrophy with mild non-specific inflammatory changes.

Examination

Length, 60.7 cm (<3rd centile).
Weight, 4.4 kg (<3rd centile).
Pyrexial, 38.3 °C (axilla).
Mildly dehydrated.
Pulse, 108 beats/min.
Heart sounds, normal.
Chest: crepitations, right upper zone.
Abdomen: distended, no tenderness, no hepatosplenomegaly, wasting of buttocks.

Investigations

Hb, 9 g/100 ml.
WBC: 10.4×10^9/litre; neutrophils, 80%; band cells, 10%; lymphocytes, 6%; monocytes, 4%.
Sodium, 130 mmol/litre.
Potassium, 3.4 mmol/litre.
Bicarbonate, 16 mmol/litre.
Urea, 9.2 mmol/litre.
Calcium, 2.0 mmol/litre.
Liver function tests, normal.
MSU, no growth.
Stool culture, salmonella species.
Blood culture, no growth.
Chest X-ray, consolidation in the right-upper and middle lobes.
Chromosome analysis: failed due to poor mitosis.

Questions

1. What is the most important investigation to carry out at this stage?
2. What two aspects of treatment for this acute episode would you concentrate on at first?
3. What diagnosis would explain his recurrent problems?

Case 59

A 5-month-old male infant was admitted to the paediatric ward with difficulty in breathing. He had begun to cough 2 days previously and started sneezing the day before admission. He was breastfed but was unable to finish his feeds because of dyspnoea. On examination he had signs of an upper respiratory tract infection and was treated effectively with 0.5% ephedrine nose drops before feeds. It was then noticed that he had yellow-tinged sclerae. His urine contained no bilirubin and his stools were not pale. Examination demonstrated mild icterus, hepatomegaly to 4 cm below the costal margin but no splenomegaly. Weight, 6.6 kg (25th centile).

Investigations

Bilirubin: 140 μmol/litre, 80 μmol/litre conjugated.
AST, 110 iu/litre.
Alkaline phosphatase, 140 iu/litre.
  The obstetric notes were reviewed. He was born at term, after an uneventful pregnancy, birth weight 3.17 kg. He became mildly jaundiced on day 3, serum bilirubin 180 μmol/litre, conjugated 40 μmol/litre. He was discharged on day 7 with no further investigation. He had fed well at home and had gained weight, albeit slowly.
  Following the initial post-admission investigations subsequent results revealed:
Bilirubin: 170 μmol/litre, 140 μmol/litre conjugated.
AST, 150 iu/litre.
5-Nucleotidase, 30 iu/litre.
Alkaline phosphatase, 190 iu/litre.
Treponema pallidum fluorescent antibody titre (FAT), negative.
Blood cultures × 3, negative.
Antibody titres to: rubella, 1:8; CMV, 1:8; toxoplasmosis, 1:8; herpes virus 1:8.
Reducing substances in stool and urine, negative.
Ultrasound demonstrated an enlarged liver with no other delineated lesion.
  The liver enlarged further without concomitant splenomegaly;

the urine became dark and contained bilirubin, the stools became pale and putty-like. Liver biopsy; occasional giant cells, proliferation of bile ductules, inflammatory cell infiltrate.

Questions

1. Give two possible diagnoses.

Case 60

A 3-year-old boy is admitted with a 4-day history of general malaise with dark urine. He had been fit and healthy previously. Twenty-four hours prior to admission he had become jaundiced with itching associated with anorexia and nausea. There had been no change of stool colour and no other symptoms of note. In the past there was no history of consequence and all immunizations had been given apart from pertussis. He was on no medication. The mother was Iraqi and the father Egyptian. There was one 5-year-old female sibling who was well, and they had lived in the UK for several years.

Examination

Height, 87.2 cm (3rd centile).
Weight, 12.9 kg (10th centile).
Miserable, afebrile.
Pale, clinically anaemic.
Marked jaundice.
Pulse, 120 beats/min; blood pressure, 80/60 mmHg.
Heart sounds, normal.
Chest, clear.
Ears and throat, normal.
Generalized lymphadenopathy.
Abdomen: liver 1 cm, palpable, non-tender; spleen, not palpable.
No abnormal neurological signs.

Investigations

Hb, 5.5 g/100 ml.
Film: fragmented RBC + + +, Heinz bodies present.
Reticulocytes, 12%.
WBC, 20.0 × 10^9/litre.
Platelets, 203 × 10^9/litre.
Urea, 4.0 mmol/litre.
Sodium, 134 mmol/litre.
Potassium, 3.8 mmol/litre.
Total protein, 58 g/litre.
Australia antigen, negative.

Questions

1. What is the diagnosis?
2. Give three further investigations you would do.
3. What are four of the most common precipitating factors?

Case 61

A 15-month-old child was seen regularly in Outpatients for recurrent chest infections. He had had several chest infections in
the first 7 months, all treated successfully by his general practitioner. However, after further episodes, he was referred to hospital.

The chest infections were neither seasonal nor preceded by an
upper respiratory tract infection. They had become less frequent
since he started walking. Each episode resolved rapidly with
antibiotic therapy, but from the age of 5 months he had had a
persistent cough and was noted to wheeze occasionally. He fed
well on a mixed diet and drank easily from a teacher beaker. His
mother noticed that he had coughing episodes sometimes whilst
drinking but he did not lose fluid though his nose. He had one or
two bowel actions daily; the stools were brown, not offensive and
flushed away easily.

He was born at 37 weeks' gestation, birth weight 2.74 kg. He
was transferred to the special care baby unit on day 3 because of

choking episodes. All investigations, including a chest X-ray, were normal and he was discharged aged 8 days. Thereafter, he still had occasional coughing episodes whilst feeding and developed his first chest infection aged 5 weeks.

He smiled at 10 weeks, sat unsupported at 7 months and walked at 12 months. He was the first-born child of 'elderly' parents. His father, aged 48 years, was a British Rail 'gang' foreman. His mother, aged 40 years, retained her job as ticket collector. They lived in a privately rented, centrally heated one-bedroomed flat; neither parent smoked.

Examination

Apyrexial.
Height, 75 cm (10th centile).
Weight, 9.5 kg (10th centile).
Pulse, 96 beats/min; sinus arrhythmia.
Heart sounds, normal.
Trachea, central.
Bilateral scattered crepitations and rhonchi in lower zones.
No hepatosplenomegaly.
Cranial nerves, intact.
Co-ordination, normal for age.
Tone, normal.
Reflexes, normal.
Plantars, downgoing.
Speech: single words used appropriately; no dribbling.

Investigations

Hb, 12.1 g/100 ml.
WBC, 7.3×10^9/litre.
IgG, 7.3 g/litre (normal range, 3.0–12.0 g/litre).
IgM, 0.7 g/litre (normal range, 0.2–1.0 g/litre).
IgA, 0.3 g/litre (normal range, 0.2–0.8 g/litre).
Sweat test, × 2: sodium, 25 mmol/litre; 21 mmol/litre.
Stool tryptic activity, detected 1 in 20.
No fat globules or meat fibres seen.
ECG, no abnormalities.
Chest X-ray, patchy shadowing both lower lobes.

Questions

1. Give two possible diagnoses.
2. Give one useful diagnostic investigation.

Case 62

A 27-year-old Latin American woman gave birth, at term, to a female infant weighing 3.75 kg. The pregnancy had been uncomplicated, labour had started spontaneously and the delivery was normal. Mother and infant were well during the immediate postnatal period, so were transferred to the ward. The infant was put to the breast immediately and suckled well. At 6 hours of life, the baby had a short apnoeic spell lasting approximately 30 s. She became centrally cyanosed during the episode, but responded to tactile stimuli rapidly. A Dextrostix taken immediately after the episode gave a reading of 0 mmol/litre. A further breast feed was given, but 15 min later the Dextrostix reading was still 0 mmol/litre. In view of the earlier symptoms, an intravenous infusion of 10% dextrose was commenced. However, after 15 min the Dextrostix reading was between 1 and 2 mmol/litre.

The mother had lived in England for the past 7 years and was married to an English journalist. There had been no episodes of illness or pyrexia during the pregnancy, or any known contact with exanthemata contacts.

The first child, born 2 years earlier, had died in the early neonatal period of unknown causes.

Examination

No dysmorphic features.
No petechiae.
No jaundice.
Cardiovascular and respiratory systems, normal.
Marked hepatosplenomegaly.
Not jittery or irritable.

Investigations

Hb, 16.7 g/100 ml.
WBC, 11.3×10^9/litre.
Blood glucose at time of first Dextrostix, 0.7 mmol/litre.
pH, 7.29.
P_{O_2}, 11.7 kPa.
P_{CO_2}, 4.8 kPa.
Bicarbonate, 15 mmol/litre.
Base excess, -9 mmol/litre.
Lumbar puncture: 12×10^6/litre RBCs; 0×10^6/litre WBCs; no organisms seen.
Bilirubin, 4 mmol/litre.

Questions

1. Give two further helpful investigations.
2. Give a possible diagnosis.

Case 63

A 7-month-old boy is sent for admission by his general practitioner. For the past 3 weeks he has had intermittent diarrhoea and vomiting with a mild pyrexia, he has been treated with clear fluids each time. The fluids were readily taken and the situation improved, but only for a few days, when the problems returned. There had been no cough or other respiratory problem.

He was born at term weighing 3.2 kg. He was breastfed and initial weight gain was thought to be satisfactory at the local baby clinic. Since 3 months of age he has had several episodes of pyrexia for which no definite cause has been found. He has been treated with antibiotics on a couple of occasions, with a slow response. He was noted to be frequently miserable, constipated, have a poor appetite, and gain weight very slowly, although still only breastfed. He has had his first triple immunization only, having been ill at other times.

The family are Caucasian and both parents are well. The father is a civil servant and the mother a housewife. There are two daughters, both alive and well.

Examination

Length, 65.1 cm (3rd centile).
Weight, 5.1 kg (<3rd centile).
Irritable.
Dehydrated with dry mouth and loss of skin turgor.
Mild pyrexia, 38 °C (rectal).
Pulse, 112 beats/min; blood pressure, 65/30 mmHg.
Heart sounds, normal.
Chest, clear.
Fauces, tympanic membranes not inflamed.
No lymphadenopathy.
Abdomen, normal.
No neurological abnormalities.

Investigations

Hb, 12.6 g/100 ml.
WBC: 11.4×10^9/litre; neutrophils, 46%; lymphocytes, 51%; mono-cytes, 2%; eosinophils., 1%.
Sodium, 167 mmol/litre.
Potassium, 4.8 mmol/litre.
Bicarbonate, 27 mmol/litre.
Urea, 7.9 mmol/litre.
Calcium, 2.4 mmol/litre.
Plasma osmolarity, 313 mosmol/litre.
Urine: micros, 3 WBC $\times 10^9$/litre; culture, no growth; ward tests, NAD.
Blood culture, no growth.
CSF: micros; no cells; culture, no growth; protein, 0.45 g/litre; sugar, 3.1 mmol/litre.

Questions

1. What is the most likely diagnosis?
2. What two additional pieces of information do you need to confirm your diagnosis?
3. What is the treatment?

Case 64

A 10-year-old boy is admitted with a 5-day history of sore throat, cough, frontal headache and posterior neck pain. He had been seen by his family doctor earlier in the week when a diagnosis of upper respiratory infection was made and co-trimoxazole prescribed. On the day before admission he was seen in Casualty in view of his lack of improvement, and changed on to erythromycin. Over the next 24 hours he had become progressively distressed with the neck pain and difficulty in breathing.

In the past he had tonsillitis at the age of 5 years but no other major problems. His mother, father and 5-year-old sister had all been well and there was no known infectious contact. They lived in a three-bedroomed council house.

Examination

Height, 143.7 cm (90th centile).
Weight, 31.3 kg (50th centile).
Pyrexial, 38.5 °C (oral).
Distressed, unable to lie down comfortably.
Pulse, 100 beats/min, regular, with volume diminution during inspiration.
Heart sounds, normal; no added sounds.
Respiratory rate, 40 breaths/min.
Breath sounds, normal; no added sounds.
No other positive signs on examination.

He was observed overnight but the following morning there was no improvement and he was still complaining bitterly of neck pain. On examination he had shallow rapid breathing and on auscultation bronchial breathing could be heard in a small area of the lower anterolateral chest on the right. There was also a rough scratching sound in time with the heart beat heard at the lower left sternal border.

Investigations

Hb, 10.8 g/100 ml.
WBC: 11.8×10^9/litre; neutrophils, 84%; lymphocytes, 13%; monocytes, 1%.
Platelets, 468×10^9/litre.

Questions

1. What is the diagnosis?
2. What are the three most likely aetiologies?
3. What are the five most important investigations you would undertake immediately?
4. What two lines of treatment would you institute?

Case 65

An 11-year-old West Indian boy was admitted unconscious to the Casualty department. He had been the victim of a school-fight in which four or five older boys had attacked him. He had been beaten to the ground and then kicked repeatedly. By the time the fight was stopped, he was unconscious. On admission to the unit he was breathing spontaneously and there was no airways obstruction. He became semi-conscious within 15 min.

He was well-known to the Casualty department as he was constantly the victim of school assaults because he was considered abnormal. The school was predominantly white.

He had had one hospital admission for treatment of acute glaucoma.

He was one of seven children; one other brother, also tall, suffered similar school brutality for identical reasons, although five of the seven children attended the school.

Examination

Height, 153 cm (>90th centile).
Badly bruised face.
Left subconjunctival haemorrhage.
Left ear contused.
Multiple abrasions: right side of face, right hemithorax, right forearm and hand.
Bruising, left hemithorax.
Simple fracture, left forearm.
Pulse, 112 beats/min; sinus arrhythmia; blood pressure, 125/90 mmHg.

Short mid systolic murmur.
Pectus excavatum.
Breath sounds, normal.
Tympanic membranes, normal.
Abdomen, soft; no guarding.
Semi-conscious–could respond to questions.
Pupils equal, reactive to light.
Fundi: small area retinal detachment, left lower temporal quadrant. Reflexes, normal.
Plantars, downgoing.
Joint movement restricted because of pain from assault.

Questions

1. Give two possible diagnoses explaining the chronic abnormalities.
2. Give the urinary abnormality in each.

Case 66

A 24-year-old mother, blood group O, rhesus positive, is delivered of her third son. At birth he is noted to have purpuric spots on the back, in the groin and on the scalp. There are no other abnormal physical signs. He is a full-term, normal delivery following an uneventful pregnancy, weighing 3.64 kg, with an Apgar score of 9 at 1 min. His two male siblings, aged 2 and 4 years, were both thrombocytopenic at birth, but now are well with normal development and are receiving no treatment.

The mother is a housewife and the father a painter and decorator. Both are Caucasian and there is no family history of note.

Initial investigations

Hb, 13.4 g/100 ml.
WBC, 19.9×10^9/litre.
Platelets, 42×10^9/litre.
Film: reduced platelets, normal appearances of RBC and WBC.

Blood group, ORh−ve.

Direct Coombs test, negative.

The following day, the platelet count is 39×10^9 cells/litre, but by the third day it has dropped to 17×10^9 cells/litre and the bilirubin level is 145 mmol/litre.

Questions

1. What is the most likely cause of the thrombocytopenia?
2. What investigation would be most helpful to prove this?
3. What two lines of treatment might you consider?

Case 67

A $5\frac{1}{2}$-year-old girl had been treated for enuresis to no avail by her general practitioner using both the buzzer system and imipramine. She was then referred to a child psychiatrist with similar lack of success over 6 months and so was referred to Paediatric Outpatients to exclude organic pathology.

She had never been dry, either by day or night. The mother had attempted toilet training from 18 months onwards and the child could void a large volume of urine voluntarily, but was damp 10 min after micturition and was persistently damp thereafter. She was unaware of passing urine constantly but had bladder sensation and micturated normally. She was continent of faeces. She had never had a urinary tract infection.

She was considered of average intelligence at school, which she disliked because of constant teasing by the other children.

She had two siblings, one aged $8\frac{1}{2}$ years, the other 3 years, both of whom were continent.

The parents had been happily married for 13 years and the family lived in a small but comfortable semi-detached house in a garden suburb.

Examination

Height, 111.7 cm (50th centile).
Weight, 19.1 kg (50th centile).

Pulse, 82 beats/min; sinus arrhythmia; blood pressure, 85/60 mmHg.
Heart sounds, normal.
Kidneys palpable, not enlarged.
External genitalia, normal.
Rectal examination, normal anal tone and reflex.
Gait, normal.
No sensory loss.
Co-ordination, good.
Reflexes, normal.
Spine, normal configuration.

Investigations

Hb, 12.3 g/100 ml.
WBC, 5.9 × 10^9/litre.
Sodium, 131 mmol/litre.
Potassium, 4.2 mmol/litre.
Glucose, 4.8 mmol/litre.
Calcium, 2.3 mmol/litre.
Urea, 2.0 mmol/litre. MSU culture × 3, negative.

Questions

1. What is the diagnosis?
2. Give one investigation to help confirm your diagnosis.

Case 68

A 10-year-old Indian girl is referred to Outpatients by her general practitioner. She has had a dry cough for 3 weeks, starting with a mild pyrexia, sore throat and headache. After 1 week there was no improvement and she had developed crepitations at the right base of the chest. She was given a week's course of amoxycillin, but there was no marked improvement so she was changed to co-trimoxazole. Four days later she developed a mild macular erythematous rash on the trunk and the co-trimoxazole was stopped. The chest signs remained unchanged: she had become anorexic and lost 1.81 kg in weight.

She had been born in India, but the family had moved to England when she was 3 years old. Her previous health was good apart from gastroenteritis aged 4 years. There are four siblings, all still living at home; the youngest is aged 5 years. They enjoy good health. The father has recently had a chest infection treated with antibiotics but is now well, working in an Indian restaurant. The mother had tuberculosis shortly after arrival in the UK and has been off treatment and well for the past 7 years. The patient has been fully immunized.

Examination

Height, 1.44 cm (25th centile).
Weight, 27.1 kg (3rd centile).
Temperature, 37.2 °C (oral).
Rash – remains of faint erythematous rash on trunk and extensor surfaces of arms, non-itchy.
Pulse, 92 beats/min; sinus arrhythmia; blood pressure, 110/65 mmHg.
Heart sounds, normal.
Respiratory rate, 40 breaths/min; no cyanosis.
Percussion, dull right base.
Crepitations, right base.
Fauces, injected.
Tympanic membranes, normal.
Small, mobile non-tender tonsillar lymph nodes.
No other positive signs.

Investigations

Hb, 11.4 g/100 ml.
WBC, 6.4×10^9/litre; neutrophils, 64%; eosinophils., 2%; lymphocytes, 30%; monocytes, 4%.
Urea, 2.3 mmol/litre.
Alkaline phosphatase, 205 iu/litre.
AST, 19 iu/litre.
ALT, 24 iu/litre.
Chest X-ray: nodular opacities in right lower zone with small right pleural effusion.

Pleural fluid: clear serous fluid; micros, 2 WBC × 10^9/litre; culture, no growth; insufficient for biochemical investigation.
Sputum: upper respiratory tract commensals only.
Mantoux test, 1 in 1000: negative.
Urinalysis, negative.

Questions

1. Give three further investigations to elucidate the diagnosis.
2. What would you prescribe for effective treatment?

Case 69

A $3\frac{1}{2}$-year-old boy was brought to Casualty by his 14-year-old sister. Both parents had full-time jobs–father was a hospital porter, mother a ward domestic–and during school holidays the younger children were looked after by the eldest daughter. All the children had been playing in the local adventure playground that morning when the $3\frac{1}{2}$-year-old began to breathe abnormally. The sister described it as wheezing. This had worsened over lunch time until the sister had become alarmed and brought him to Casualty.

She did not think that he had had any previous serious illnesses. There was no available obstetric or developmental history. The two other siblings aged 10 years and 5 years were healthy and the family lived in a three-bedroomed terraced council house.

Examination

Pyrexial, 38.6 °C (axilla).
Drooling, flushed, centrally cyanosed.
No rash.
Pulse, 132 beats/min.
No added cardiac sounds.
Inspiratory and expiratory stridor.
Respiratory rate, 50 breaths/min.

Suprasternal, sternal and subcostal recession.
Breath sounds, normal.
Restless, but appropriately responsive.

Questions

1. Give two immediate therapeutic measures.
2. Give three important investigations.

Case 70

A $6\frac{1}{2}$-year-old boy was playing football in the playground on a hot summer's day, when he suddenly collapsed and became unconscious. He remained comatose for approximately 10 min during which time he was motionless. On arrival at hospital he was conscious and complaining of a headache.

He had been previously well and was an active child, playing vigorously with his older siblings. He had never lost consciousness before and there was no family history of epilepsy or migraine.

The birth had been a normal vaginal delivery with a vertex presentation at term. Birth weight was 3.38 kg and there were no neonatal complications. His development was normal. He sat unsupported at 7 months and walked at 11 months. He had coped well during his short period at school.

He was the third child of three. His father was a statistician and his mother was a professional badminton coach. They lived in a well-appointed, four-bedroomed flat. His mother had become depressed 4 months previously and had been prescribed Motival (fluphenazine and nortriptyline).

Examination

Height, 118.3 cm (75th centile).
Weight, 18.68 kg (10th centile).
Pale, not clinically anaemic.
Pulse, 110 beats/min; sinus arrhythmia; blood pressure, 90/60 mmHg.

Apex beat, forceful, fifth interspace.
Heart sounds, soft second sound.
Harsh systolic murmur left sternal edge.
Early diastolic murmur, aortic area.
Peripheral pulses, normal.
No radiofemoral delay.
Respiratory, ENT and abdominal systems, normal,
Neurological: fully conscious, answered questions appropriately,
no nuchal rigidity.
Tone and power, normal and equal in all limbs.
Cranial nerves, normal, no photophobia.
Reflexes, normal.
Plantars, downgoing.

Investigations

Hb, 12.6 g/100 ml.
WBC, 6.7 × 10^9/litre; normal differential.
Blood sugar, 7.3 mmol/litre.
Sodium, 140 mmol/litre.
Potassium, 3.9 mmol/litre.
Calcium, 2.43 mmol/litre.
Skull X-ray, no fractures.
Chest X-ray, no cardiomegaly; lung fields, normal.
Urine and plasma toxicology screen, negative.
Urinalysis, negative.

Questions

1. Give a further vital investigation.
2. What is the most likely diagnosis?
3. Give one other useful investigation.

Case 71

A 42-year-old primigravida was admitted at term in established
labour. On vaginal examination the cervix was 5 cm dilated, but

the labour then became prolonged and the infant was born following a difficult forceps delivery. The umbilical cord was around the child's neck and required cutting before delivery. Tracheal intubation with IPPV was required for 5 min, after which the infant breathed spontaneously. He was noted to be mildly cyanosed; this was presumed to be traumatic cyanosis following the difficult delivery. Nevertheless, he was admitted to the special care baby unit for observation.

The mother had attended antenatal clinic erratically, had refused all medication and continued to smoke approximately 15 cigarettes and consume at least half a bottle of wine daily. She had continued working as the editor of a well-known periodical until 38 weeks' gestation. Her husband, aged 34 years, was a reporter for a daily tabloid. They lived in a luxurious penthouse flat.

Examination

Birth weight, 2.18 kg (<3rd centile).
Traumatic cyanosis.
Pulse, 140 beats/min; blood pressure, 80/30 mmHg.
Heart sounds, thought to be normal.
Systolic murmur maximal in pulmonary area.
Pulses, bounding.
Respiratory rate, 34 breaths/min.
Chest sounds, normal. Liver, 1 cm, soft.
Neurological system, normal.

A provisional diagnosis of a patent ductus arteriosus was made and an infusion of indomethacin commenced. The infant rapidly became intensely cyanosed. The infusion was stopped and the child was transferred in oxygen to the intensive care baby unit at the nearby teaching hospital.

Examination

Deep central cyanosis.
Pulse, 163 beats/min; blood pressure, 70/30 mmHg.
Heart sounds: first sound, soft; second sound, single.
Mid systolic murmur in pulmonary area.

Investigations

ECG: sinus rhythm; axis, +110°; left ventricular dominance in precordial leads.
Chest X-ray; no cardiomegaly, oligaemic lung fields.
The child was commenced on prostaglandin and rapidly became less cyanosed.

Questions

1. What is the most likely diagnosis?
2. Give two further useful investigative techniques.

Case 72

Sammie was referred to Outpatients at the age of 14 years with a proven urinary tract infection. IVP demonstrated a normal urinary tract, but moderate constipation. Her parents had divorced when she was 9 years old. When 11 years old she sustained a head injury with loss of consciousness, post-traumatic amnesia and vomiting which neccesitated admission. Six months later she presented with a 2-week history of headaches, polyuria and polydipsia; a diagnosis of diabetes mellitus was made. She was admitted for stabilization which was rapidly achieved on twice-daily Humulin M3. Following discharge she required minor insulin adjustments to control hypoglycaemia. Shortly after this she enjoyed a happy Christmas and her mother remarried in the New Year.

Three months after diagnosis she developed simple absences, lasting up to 30 s, occurring three to four times daily. She would suddenly stop her activity, remain motionless and then resume activity with no apparent memory of the event. One such episode was witnessed in Outpatients and she was commenced on sodium valproate 20 mg/kg/day on clinical grounds. One week later she was admitted with an increasing frequency of the absences which were now lasting up to 10 min.

Obstetric history had been unremarkable, as was her developmental history. She had only received two combined immunizations as she had had a severe generalized reaction to the second one. She now attended a public day school and was academically gifted. She had recently been given her own pony. Her mother and younger sister had suffered from recurrent febrile fits in childhood. Her father had been killed in a road traffic accident some 3 years earlier.

Questions

1. What investigation is required?
2. What is the most likely diagnosis?
3. What treatment can be offered for this problem?

Case 73

An 8-month-old child was referred to Outpatients with a history of swellings in the neck for 2 weeks, persistent diarrhoea for 1 week with failure to thrive and listlessness for a protracted, but indeterminate time. His appetite had been good until the appearance of the neck swellings. He was on a normal mixed diet and pasteurized milk.

At 8 weeks old he had suffered from *Haemophilus influenzae* meningitis. This responded well to antibiotics and no neurological sequelae were detected. He had also suffered from two short episodes of gastroenteritis, both of which responded to clear fluids. He was developmentally normal and had been fully immunized.

The pregnancy had been normal, culminating in a spontaneous vertex delivery at term, birth weight 3.29 kg. He was the first-born child of East African parents. His mother had been born in the UK and neither she nor the child had ever been abroad. His father had made occasional trips back to the family business in East Africa. The company had, however, recently been liquidated; they had defaulted on their mortgage repayments, the flat had been repossessed and they were living in a squat with several other families and assorted animals.

Examination

Length, 68 cm (25th centile).
Weight 7.05 kg (3rd centile).
Head circumference, 45.4 cm (50th centile).
Pyrexial, 38.8 °C.
Respiratory rate, 70 breaths/min.
Clinically apparent wasting of the buttocks.
Generalized lymphadenopathy with hepatosplenomegaly.
   A clinical diagnosis of acute lymphoblastic leukaemia was made.

Investigations

Hb, 9.7 g/100 ml.
WBC, 13.1×10^9/litre; neutrophils 43%; lymphocytes 52%; monocytes 3%; eosinophils. 1%; basophils 1%; no blast cells.
Platelets, 263×10^9/litre.
Blood cultures, urine culture, stool culture, negative.
AST 73 iu/litre.
ALT 32 iu/litre.
SBR 29 μmol/litre.
IgG 36.1 g/litre.
IgM 1.6 g/litre.
IgA 1.3 g/litre.
   He was treated empirically with broad-spectrum antibiotics with an appparent systemic response, but no improvement in the organomegaly, lymphadenopathy, diarrhoea or tachypnoea.

Questions

1. Give two further important investigations.
2. Give two possible diagnoses.
3. What is the most likely cause of his respiratory sign?

Case 74

A 2-day-old female infant is transferred from the postnatal wards with vomiting, plus two twitching episodes, lasting 30 sec., and

2 min. Thirty minutes later she had a cyanotic attack. On admission to Special Care she had a 6 min jerking episode. BM stix was unrecordable.

She is the first child of an unrelated couple; father is a telephone sales clerk and mother a computer operator. She was born at term by normal delivery, Apgar scores 8 at 1 min and 10 at 5 min. No resuscitation was required; birth weight was 3.24 kg.

Breastfeeding had been started immediately after birth, but the baby had vomited despite two stomach washouts and later a trial of formula baby milk.

Examination

Temperature, 37.2 °C.
Ill-looking baby, irritable; high pitched cry.
Mild jaundice.
Generalized hypertonia but good sucking reflex.
Respiratory rate, 40 breaths/min.
Chest, clinically clear.
Heart rate, 130 beats/min, regular.
Heart sounds normal; no murmur heard.
Femorals, easily palpable.
Abdomen distended, slightly tender with active bowel sounds.

Investigations

On admission:
Hb 13.7 g/dl.
WBC, 11.1×10^9/litre.
Platelets, 149×10^9/litre.
Sodium, 137 mmol/litre.
Potassium, 5.5 mmol/litre.
Chloride, 100 mmol/litre.
Bicarbonate, 10.2 mmol/litre.
Urea, 11.4 mmol/litre.
Creatinine, 175 μmol/litre.
Glucose, 5.5 mmol/litre, after intravenous dextrose.
Calcium, 1.32 mmol/litre.
Albumin, 40 g/litre.
Bilirubin, 91 μmol/litre.

Arterial blood gases, pH 7.4; P_{CO_2}, 2.7 kPa, P_{O_2} 12.6 kPa, bicarbonate, 12.5 mmol/litre, base excess, -10.
CSF protein, unsuitable as heavily blood-stained.
CSF glucose, 4.0 mmol/litre.
CSF micros–RBC, 50 000/cm^3; WBC, 18 × 10^9/litre; neutrophils 50%; monocytes 50%; no growth on culture.
Urine–microscopy, NAD; culture, no growth.
Blood culture, *Streptococcus mitus* and *Neisseria* spp; Contaminants.

Initial treatment was given with intravenous dextrose, albumin, calcium, antibiotics and a loading dose of phenobarbitone. Her general condition improved; she was noted to have loose stools and be passing urine well. Repeat electrolytes the next day were as follows:
Sodium, 128 mmol/litre.
Potassium, 4.6 mmol/litre.
Chloride, 98 mmol/litre.
Bicarbonate, 10.8 mmol/litre.
Urea, 15.2 mmol/litre.
Creatinine, 141 μmol/litre.
Calcium, 1.95 mmol/litre.

The baby was restarted on a baby milk formula, but again became irritable with a tense abdomen; the loose stools continued.

Renal ultrasound, normal.
Head ultrasound, normal.
Serum lactate, 2.45 mmol/litre (normal range, 0.63–2.44).
Plasma ammonia, 63 μmol/litre (normal range, less than 55 μmol/litre).
Urinary amino acids, normal.
Bilirubin, 23 μmol/litre.
AST, 55 iu/litre.
Gamma glutamyl transferase, 117 iu/litre.
Alkaline phosphatase, 122 iu/litre.
Sodium, 135 mmol/litre.
Potassium, 4.3 mmol/litre.
Chloride, 108 mmol/litre.
Bicarbonate, 7.0 mmol/litre.
Urea, 16.2 mmol/litre.
Calcium, 1.66 mmol/litre.
Abdominal X-ray, gas noted in stomach, small and large bowel.
No evidence of obstruction, ileus or perforation.

Questions

1. What is the most likely diagnosis?
2. What simple test would you do to support this diagnosis?

Case 75

A six-year old girl is admitted from Outpatients for investigation and treatment of recurrent chest infections resistant to successive courses of antibiotics. She has severe bilateral sensorineural hearing loss, wears hearing aids and attends a special school for hearing-impaired children.

She was born at 38 weeks' gestation. Pregnancy was uncomplicated until the third trimester when there was increasing hypertension. Labour was induced, delivery was by forceps and the birth weight was 2.9 kg. The baby was admitted to Special Care with 'breathing problems' and diagnosed as having pneumonia. She was discharged home on day 10 on no treatment.

During the first year, she was always snuffly, and after that she had the normal number of coughs and colds. Aged 4 years it was noted she had severe catarrh; she was given a sinus washout and since then had been much better. Aged 5 years, just before starting school, each cold 'went to her chest' and was associated with wheezing. Over the past year she had had a chest infection requiring antibiotics virtually every 2 weeks. The most recent episode had not cleared despite several courses of antibiotics.

In the family, mother is single, living with her parents, and working in a factory during the day. She had asthma for the first time 2 years ago; her sister and niece also suffered from asthma and eczema.

Examination

Height, 107 cm (10th centile).
Weight, 22 kg (75th centile).
No cyanosis, no tachypnoea.
Early finger clubbing.

Tympanic membranes both dull and retracted with old healing perforation on the left.

Throat, not inflamed.

Chest–normal shape, percussion note very dull left base with bronchial breathing on auscultation. Scattered crepitations and rhonchi in all other areas of the chest.

Pulses, normal.

Blood pressure, 100/60 mmHg.

Heart sounds normal, no murmur.

Abdomen–liver, kidneys, spleen impalpable, no masses felt.

CNS, bilateral deafness, no other abnormality found.

Investigations

Hb 12.3 g/100 ml.

WBC, 19.9×10^9/litre; neutrophils, 62%; lymphocytes, 32%; monocytes, 6%.

Platelets, 731×10^9/litre.

ESR, 29 mm/h.

Urea and electrolytes, normal.

Liver function tests, normal.

Protein electrophoresis, diffuse increase in gamma globulin band.

IgG, 12.5 g/litre (normal range, 4.6–12.4 g/litre).

IgA, 1.6 g/litre (normal range, 0.3–1.5 g/litre).

IgM, 1.1 g/litre (normal range, 0.4–2.0 g/litre).

Free thyroxine 14.1 pmol/litre (normal range, 8.0–24.0 pmol/litre).

Sweat osmolality, 83 mmol/kg (normal range, 62–139 mmol/kg).

Sputum, purulent; culture, *Haemophilus influenzae*.

Chest X-ray–collapse consolidation left lower lobe with mediastinal shift to the left; patchy consolidation in the right lower lobe; some collapse of lung adjacent to the horizontal fissure.

Sinus X-rays, no definite abnormality seen.

Postnasal space X-rays, slight adenoidal enlargement but the airway is satisfactory.

Questions

1. What is the diagnosis?
2. What are the two most likely causes?
3. What two investigations would you perform?

Case 76

An 11-month-old boy is admitted with a history of poor feeding for the past week, mild pyrexia and poor weight gain over the past 3–4 weeks. He was born at term by normal delivery; his birth weight was on the 25th centile. He was breastfed for 3 months, then changed to baby formula milk and weaned from 4 months of age. Mother was a good attender at the local baby clinic; all immunizations had been given; he passed the 6-week check; weight gain had been satisfactory and development normal for age. He is the second child in the family; the first, a boy aged 5 years is in good health. There is no family history of note. Mother has just started part-time work as a receptionist, father teaches the technical aspects of photography.

Examination

Pale.
Temperature, 38.2 °C.
No lymphadenopathy.
Pulses all present, good volume.
Heart sounds, grade 2 systolic murmur heard at the lower left sternal border and apex.
Chest, clear.
Liver, 2 cm below the costal margin, spleen tipped.
Throat and tympanic membranes, not inflamed.

Investigations

Hb, 5.3 g/100 ml.
MCV, 83 fl; MCHC, 33 g/dl; reticulocytes, 2.4%.
WBC, 12.5×10^9/litre; neutrophils 60%; lymphocytes 32%; monocytes 5%; eosinophils 2%.
Platelets, 105×10^9/litre.
Prothrombin time, 14 s; control, 13 s.
APTT, 37 s; control, 35 s.
Sodium, 135 mmol/litre.
Potassium, 4.2 mmol/litre.
Chloride, 102 mmol/litre.
Bicarbonate, 19 mmol/litre.

Urea, 6.1 mmol/litre.

Total bilirubin, 16 μmol/litre.

AST, 45 iu/litre.

Gamma glutamyl transferase, 60 iu/litre.

Alkaline phosphatase, 189 iu/litre.

Albumin, 36 g/litre.

Calcium, 2.2 mmol/litre.

Blood culture after 2 days' incubation grew *Moraxella* spp. from both bottles; ?Contaminant.

Urine microscopy–5 WBC $\times$ 10^6/litre; 5 RBC $\times$ 10^6/litre.

Culture, no growth.

C-reactive protein, 126 mg/litre.

The child was given a blood transfusion and amoxycillin. Three days later he had improved quite markedly, but the murmur was still present. He was discharged home to finish the course of antibiotics. Ten days later he was brought back into Casualty in a collapsed state.

Question

1. What is the most likely diagnosis?

2 Answers and discussions

Case 1

Answers

1. (a) Sickle cell anaemia.
   (b) Septic arthritis.
   (c) Pauciarticular juvenile chronic arthritis.
   (d) Rheumatic fever.
   (e) Ulcerative colitis.
   (f) Henoch-Schönlein purpura.
2. (a) Haemoglobin electrophoresis.
   (b) Aspiration of the joint space.
   (c) Anti-streptolysin O titre.
   (d) Blood cultures.
   (e) Erythrocyte sedimentation rate.
   (f) Plasma viscosity.
   (g) C-reactive protein.
   (h) Anti-staphylococcal lysins.

Discussion

This child is West Indian and presents with anaemia and a monoarticular arthritis of a large joint. The first diagnosis should, therefore, be sickle cell disease. Homozygous sickle cell disease often presents in the first year of life as fetal haemoglobin concentration decreases; however, there is a spectrum of severity, including haemoglobin C and D disease, so initial presentation at this age is feasible. Haemoglobin electrophoresis is, therefore, indicated.

Sickle cell disease may produce protean orthopaedic problems. Presentation in the first year of life; dactylitis of hands or feet is pathognomonic. Thereafter any bone may be affected by a sickling crisis with capillary thrombosis and subsequent infarction. Involvement of the femoral head may lead to aseptic necrosis, and large areas of destruction in the long bones may produce subsequent deformity. Other areas of deformity include the skull, with bossing and widening of the medulla caused by marrow extension. Osteomyelitis can be difficult to differentiate as clinical signs are similar and X-ray changes occur late.

Septic arthritis, although now no longer common, is still a potential complication of any bacteraemia. Many organisms have been implicated, but staphylococcal infection is commonly recognized. The effect of septic arthritis is dependent on age. In the first year of life nutrient arteries pass through the metaphysis to the epiphysis, allowing bacterial extension and sepsis. There is rapid destruction of the joint, but X-ray changes occur late. In contrast, X-ray changes may occur within a few days in the older child; also, the epiphysis is protected by a metaphyseal plate. Aspiration of the joint spaces produces a purulent fluid with a high neutrophil count ($>50\,000$ mm^{-3}) with low glucose concentration. Gram's staining should identify an organism. Prolonged antibiotic therapy is indicated.

The classification of childhood arthritis is still not uniformly accepted: juvenile chronic arthritis is used in Europe, juvenile arthritis is utilized worldwide. There is further classification based on the number of joints involved. Pauciarticular arthritis (affecting four joints or less for 3 months) is the commonest presentation. Type I mainly affects girls between 1 and 5 years. Rheumatoid factor is negative, but approximately 60% of patients carry antinuclear factor, which has a close correlation with chronic iridocyclitis. There is also an association with human leukocyte antigen (HLA) A2 DR5 and DRw8. HLA B27 is associated with the type II pauciarticular type. This mainly affects older boys and is frequently associated with the later development of sacroiliitis. Orthopaedic problems include periostitis, joint destruction with subsequent limitation of movement, bony erosions and osteoporosis. Polyarticular arthritis (five or more joints affected for 3 months) is divided by IgM RF. RF tends to be negative in children younger than 6 years old and associated with DRw8. Rheumatoid-positive disease occurs in the older age group, associated with DR4. Systemic disease is characterized by a swinging pyrexia, spiking twice daily, an evanescent pink maculopapular rash, lymphadenopathy, splenomegaly and hepatomegaly. Echocardiography reveals a 30% incidence of pericarditis. The progress of the disease may be followed by sequential measurement of the ESR or C-reactive protein.

Rheumatic fever is a possible, albeit rare, diagnosis despite the absence of a preceding illness. Evidence of recent streptococcal infection would be afforded by a raised ASOT or other anti-strep-tococcal antibodies. Diagnosis is largely clinical and depends on a combination of major and minor signs. Major manifestations are carditis, polyarthritis, chorea, erythema marginatum and sub-cutaneous nodules; minor manifestations include fever, arthralgia, raised ESR or acute-phase proteins, leukocytosis and a prolonged P–R interval. Diagnosis is confirmed if the patient has one sign from both categories plus a supporting third manifestation. The arthritis of rheumatic fever may initially mimic septic arthritis, but then becomes flitting, with other joints being affected every 2–3 days. Treatment is with antibiotics, anti-inflammatory agents and possibly steroids. The length of bed rest is dependent on the severity of the carditis.

Ulcerative colitis or regional enteritis may produce clinically identical arthritis. Usually only a few joints are involved and the arthritis occurs when the enteric disease is active. However, the child is anaemic and ulcerative colitis can present as an arthritis alone with no bowel symptoms. The prognosis for joint function in either disease is excellent.

Further reading

Ansell, B. A. (1990). Classification and nomenclature. In *Paediatric Rheumatology Update*, Ed. by P. Woo, P. H. White, B. A. Ansell, p. 3. (Oxford; Oxford University Press)

Ansell, B. A. (1990). Overall review. In *Paediatric Rheumatology Update*, Ed. by P. Woo, P. H. White, B. A. Ansell, p. 133. (Oxford; Oxford University Press)

Sickle cell anaemia

Bennett, O. M. (1990) Bone and joint manifestations of sickle cell anaemia. *Journal of Bone and Joint Surgery* **72**:494–9.

Case 2

Answers

1. (a) Visual field testing.
   (b) Lateral X-ray of the skull.
   (c) Assessment of hypothalamopituitary axis with clonidine or insulin tolerance test and thyrotrophin releasing hormone/luteinizing hormone-releasing hormone (TRH/LHRH) injection.

(d) Thyroxine.
(e) CT scan.
(f) Bone age.
(g) Testicular responsiveness to three injections of human chorionic gonadotrophin.

Discussion

This boy presents two major problems–small stature and delayed puberty–which are interrelated. The most common problem is constitutional pubertal and growth delay. This normally results when a child, generally a boy, has been growing along the 10th centile and continuation of the prepubertal growth rate into the teen years results in a drop to below the third centile. There may be a similar pattern in other members of the family, and quite often the testes will have begun to increase in size, even though there are no other secondary sexual characteristics apparent. Neither of these points are true in this case. Chronic illness such as asthma, Crohn's disease and anorexia nervosa are also causes, but again cannot be blamed here. Very occasionally hypopituitarism is the problem.

In boys and girls, 97% show signs of puberty by their 14th birthday. In boys it is reasonable to wait until their 15th birthday, but then delayed puberty should be investigated. Delayed puberty can be due to hypothalamic, pituitary, gonadal and adrenal causes, apart from constitutional reasons.

This boy probably has multiple pituitary hormone deficiencies since short stature is a prominent feature. In isolated gonadotrophin deficiency the patients may be of normal stature or even tall for their age. Anterior pituitary deficiencies relate to the following factors:

1. Congenital–genetic, midline embryonic defects or haemorrhagic infarction at birth.
2. Acquired–space-occupying lesions, post-injury or surgery, post-irradiation, temporary failure due to emotional deprivation or hypothyroidism.

A space-occupying lesion is high on the list here in the region of the hypothalamus/pituitary in view of the morning headaches suggestive of raised intracranial pressure and the previously probably normal growth and development. Investigations should be aimed at simple preliminary tests, i.e. visual field tests and lateral X-rays of the skull to view the pituitary fossa, clinoid processes and presence or absence of calcification. Hypothyroidism due to thyroid disease should be ruled out by doing triiodothyronine and thyroxine estimations.

After this, an assessment of the hypothalamus–pituitary–target-organ axis should be conducted, including an insulin tolerance test with TRH/LHRH stimulation and measuring the glucose, cortisols, growth hormone, prolactin, thyrotrophin stimulating hormone, luteinizing hormone (LH), follicle-stimulating hormone (FSH) and thyroxine values regularly.

To complete the assessment bone age should be done. This would be expected to be delayed in both constitutional small stature and growth hormone deficiency and thus would mainly be helpful in prognosticating growth potential. A CT scan would help in identifying the position and size of a space-occupying lesion. Lastly, testicular responsiveness can be tested to three injections of human chorionic gonadotrophin if stimulation is in doubt after the hypothalamus–pituitary–target-organ axis test. Chronically understimulated testes may take longer to respond.

Further reading

Cuttler, L. (1987). Evaluation of growth disorders in children. *Pediatrician*, **14**, 109–20.

Mahoney, C. P. (1987). Evaluating the child with short stature. *Pediatric Clinics of North America*, **34**, 825–49.

Stanhope, R. and Brook, C. G. D. (1989). Disorders of puberty. In *Clinical Paediatric Endocrinology*, Ed. by C. G. D. Brook, pp. 200–8. (Oxford; Blackwell Scientific Publications)

Case 3

Answers

1. Perthes disease.
2. (a) Tuberculous arthritis.
   (b) Transient synovitis of the hip, especially after streptococcal infections.
   (c) Juvenile chronic arthritis.

(d) Osteoid osteoma.
3. Healing in 2–3 years.

Discussion

Perthes disease is an ischaemic necrosis of the upper femoral epiphysis which presents with persistent or variable pain in the hip, often associated with some degree of pain in the groin and knee in a previously healthy child. The commonest ages of presentation are between 4 and 9 years and boys are affected four times as commonly as girls. On examination the child is usually limping with physical signs limited to the affected hip, with some loss of movement, particularly in flexion, abduction and internal rotation. X-ray changes depend on the stage of the disease. Initially there is a destructive phase where sclerosis is the first radiographic change in the affected head, representing dead bone. Diffuse rarefaction of the entire femur may occur. As repair occurs and dead tissue is replaced by fibrous tissue, there will be both radiolucent and sclerotic shadows with fragmentation of the femoral head which becomes smaller and flatter. The femoral head will then gradually enlarge as the femoral ossification centre enlarges and the femoral neck widens, following repair of destructive foci in both the head and metaphysis.

A technetium-99 scan will show decreased uptake over the femoral head since it is avascular and the isotope is used to show 'hot spots' with increased blood supply. The surrounding zone of increased uptake represents some revascularization and repair. Magnetic resonance imaging (MRI) scan has recently been shown to be extremely sensitive in demonstrating changes in Perthes disease. Haematological examination is usually normal, but in this case worsening of the condition appears to have been started by upper respiratory tract infections, with a slightly raised ESR. There is a condition of recurrent transient synovitis of the hip following mild episodes of streptococcal infections, where the degree of loss of movement in the hip will vary from acute spasm with loss of all movement to mild restriction. There is no muscle wasting. Transient synovitis of unknown aetiology also occurs and occasionally Perthes disease appears to follow such an episode. Radiologically there is usually no abnormality in transient synovitis, although there may be slight widening of the joint space on the affected side.

Tuberculous arthritis usually causes insidious monoarticular arthritis of the knee, hip or wrist. Pain is the usual symptom, together with marked swelling of the affected joint and localized muscle wasting. General health may not be good, with low-grade pyrexia, weight loss and possibly some other site of infection causing symptoms. Osteoporosis is the earliest X-ray finding and is followed by erosive changes. Thus the picture presented here is not typical either in symptomatology or in findings.

Juvenile chronic arthritis can present as a monoarticular arthritis usually of knee, ankle or wrist. However, the radiological findings are of osteoporosis in the early stages followed by accelerated epiphyseal maturation. There is boggy soft tissue swelling of the joint, sometimes with constitutional upset and occasionally positive antinuclear antibodies. These findings do not fit with the case outlined above.

Osteoid osteoma when placed near a joint can present with acute or subacute recurrent loss of movement. It particularly affects the trochanteric area, thus hip problems are common. Radiologically it can be difficult to detect, but widespread osteoporosis and local sclerosis are found and thus could be a possibility here, although most unlikely.

Other benign bone cysts can mimic arthritis; malignancies can give a mixed osteolytic and sclerotic picture. However, the history in this case makes malignancy unlikely.

The prognosis in Perthes disease is usually good, with gradual healing over 2–3 years.

Further reading

Bohr, H. H. (1980). Development and course. *Clinical Orthopaedics and Related Research*, **150**, 3–35.

Calve, J. (1980). The classic. On a particular form of pseudo-coxalgia associated with a characteristic deformity of the upper end of the femur. *Clinical Orthopaedics and Related Research*, **150**, 2–35.

Fisher, R. L. *et al.* (1980). Isotopic bone imaging. *Clinical Orthopaedics and Related Research*, **150**, 23–29.

Gershwin, D. H. (1980). Evaluation and prognosis in Legg–Calve–Perthes' disease. *Clinical Orthopaedics and Related Research*, **150**, 16–21.

Lloyd-Roberts, G. C. and Fixsen, J. (1990). *Orthopaedics in Infancy and Childhood*, pp. 147–62. (Oxford; Butterworth-Heinemann)

Silverman, F. N. and Kuhn, J. P. (1990). *Essentials of Caffey's Paediatric X-ray Diagnosis. Part VI. The Limbs and Pelvis*, pp. 735–1016. (Chicago; Year Book Medical Publishers)

Wynne-Davies, R. (1980). Some etiologic factors in Perthes' disease. *Clinical Orthopaedics and Related Research*, **150**, 12–15.

Case 4

Answers

1. (a) Urea/creatinine.
   (b) Serum and urine osmolality.
   (c) Blood glucose.
   (d) Urine microscopy and culture.
   (e) Urinary calcium.
2. Psychogenic polydipsia.

Discussion

This child presents with polydipsia and polyuria, diffuse abdominal pain, a dying father and failing school standards. Possible diagnoses include diabetes mellitus, chronic renal failure, diabetes insipidus and psychogenic polydipsia.

Diabetes mellitus is unlikely because of the absence of glycosuria, but blood glucose concentration must be measured. Childhood diabetes usually presents acutely with dehydration and ketoacidosis.

Chronic renal failure causes polyuria with low urine osmolality secondary to tubular damage, with a poor response to antidiuretic hormone (ADH). This may also be induced by hypokalaemia, hypercalcaemia or by renal infections. Both electrolytes mentioned have normal values and there is no history of episodes of weakness suggestive of periodic hypokalaemia. There is no history of overt renal or urinary tract infections, her blood pressure is normal, she is on the 25th centile for both height and weight and the tubules are capable of responding to ADH. Chronic renal failure is, therefore, unlikely. Diabetes insipidus is either hypothalamic or nephrogenic in origin. Nephrogenic diabetes insipidus is sex-linked recessive and is, therefore, confined to males. However, there are individual cases of affected females and some female heterozygotes may demonstrate impaired concentrating ability. Nephrogenic diabetes insipidus usually presents in infancy, but later onset can occur. Symptoms include dehydration, fever, failure to thrive, vomiting and constipation. Mental retardation may be induced. The lesion appears due to end-organ failure rather than the production of an abnormal hormone, or rapid inactivation. Treatment is with thiazide diuretics which are thought to act by inducing sodium depletion with subsequent increased sodium resorption in the proximal tubules with antidiuretic effect.

Differentiation between hypothalamic and nephrogenic diabetes insipidus is achieved by administering ADH, which produces a concentrated urine in those with a hypothalamic lesion. Also the urine osmolality in hypothalamic diabetes insipidus is generally between 50 and 200 mosmol/litre, whereas that in nephrogenic diabetes is between 80 and 120 mosmol/litre.

Hypothalamic diabetes insipidus and psychogenic polydipsia are differentiated by the water deprivation test. If the problem is psychogenic, urine osmolality should reach 869–1309 mosmol/litre; however, if the problem is long-standing, there may be inadequate response to ADH with poor concentrating ability.

The urine may become more concentrated during dehydration in hypothalamic diabetes insipidus, but can only reach a maximum of 285 mosmol/litre, which excludes the diagnosis in this case. An alternative differentiating investigation is to infuse hypertonic sodium chloride. In normal children, a urine of smaller volume and greater osmolality will be passed. Those with hypothalamic diabetes insipidus will show neither change. In this case, with poor concentration it would be reasonable to repeat the water deprivation test.

Hypothalamic diabetes insipidus may be either idiopathic, which is more common, or secondary to local pathology. These disorders include intracranial tumours–such as craniopharyngioma, optic glioma, and Langerhans-cell histiocytosis (histiocytosis X)–encephalitis and severe head injury. Rarer causes include toxoplasmosis, leukaemia and cerebral haemorrhage. Investigations will be directed towards differentiating these causes. The inheritance of idiopathic hypothalamic diabetes insipidus is sporadic, autosomal dominant or sex-linked recessive. Treatment is with the synthetic arginine ADH desaminocys-d-arginine-8-vasopressin (ADH DDAVP).

Psychogenic polydipsia is the most likely diagnosis in this child. She presents with vague diffuse abdominal pain, her adoptive father is dying and her school performance is suffering. She has reduced concentrating ability but is able to produce a urine of greater osmolality than is possible in diabetes insipidus. Psychogenic polydipsia is a symptom of a plethora of emotional disturbances and treatment is either individual or family psychotherapy.

Further reading

Savage, J. M. (1986). Polyuria and polydipsia. In *Clinical Paediatric Nephrology*, Ed. by R. J. Postlethaite, pp. 98–101. (Bristol; Wright)

de Wardener, H. E. (ed) (1985). The Kidney, 5th edn. pp. 307–14. (London; Churchill Livingstone)

Case 5

Answers

1. Lead encephalopathy.
2. (a) Encephalitis, viral.
   (b) Space-occupying lesion.
   (c) Meningitis–particularly tuberculous.
   (d) Drug intoxication.
3. (a) CT scan or MRI scan.
   (b) Blood lead level.
   (c) Urinary coproporphyrins.
   (d) Full blood count with film for basophilic stippling.
   (e) X-rays of long bones and abdomen.
   (f) Urine: amino acid chromatography and glucose content.
   (g) Plasma phosphate level.
   (h) Urine for toxicology.

Discussion

Lead encephalopathy is one of the rare but well-recognized causes of coma and convulsions in a child. It should be included in the differential diagnosis of anaemia, convulsions, mental retardation and severe behavioural disorders. Lead poisoning is more common amongst lower-income groups and occurs most frequently in children who live in old houses where there may be lead-containing paint, especially in those children with pica. Young children absorb a higher percentage of lead from their gut than adults and retain more. Studies in young growing animals have shown that diets high in fat and low in calcium, iron and other minerals increase the absorption of lead, and this type of diet is again more prevalent in poor-income families.

This child appears to have undergone a normal delivery with mainly normal milestones. However, sitting unsupported late at 10 months and only babbling and cooing at 8 months could suggest a degree of neglect on the parents' part. This is further confirmed by the lack of visits to a baby clinic and the failure to thrive. Persistent pica is associated with inadequate mothering.

The presence and severity of symptoms depend upon the amount of lead ingested and the frequency of pica. The earliest symptoms are hyperirritability associated with lethargy and anorexia. Sporadic vomiting, abdominal pain and constipation are manifestations of lead colic but are not mentioned in this child. Loss of recently acquired development skills may occur and anaemia is characteristic. Thus behavioural changes can precede insomnia and headaches which frequently herald the onset of lead encephalopathy with convulsions, impairment of consciousness, persistent vomiting and ataxia. Massive cerebral oedema is present, although the classic signs of papilloedema and cracked-pot sound on percussion of the skull may not be present. Peripheral neuropathy is uncommon in the young child but may develop and particularly affects the dorsiflexors of the wrist and feet. Acute lead poisoning may cause a Fanconi type of proximal tubular damage with generalized aminoaciduria, glycosuria and hyperphosphaturia. Hypertension has been reported.

Lead poisoning can also take a more chronic course with recurrent symptomatic episodes which abate spontaneously. In the past up to 45% of mentally retarded children have been reported as having high blood lead levels. Whether this is cause or effect is not known. There is no definite blood lead level when a child becomes symptomatic; it varies considerably from approximately 60 μg/100 ml to 250 μg/100 ml. However, in lead encephalopathy the blood level usually exceeds 100 μg/100 ml.

Other tests which should be employed in an emergency to make a diagnosis are:

1. A strongly positive qualitative urinary coproporphyrin test.
2. Microcytic hypochromic anaemia with punctate basophilia or stippled erythroblasts in the bone marrow.
3. Radiopaque flecks in the intestine indicating recent ingestion of lead-containing material. Lines of increased density at the metaphyses of long bones.
4. Urine tests for amino acids and glucose levels, together with hypophosphataemia.

Other abnormalities include increased δ-aminolaevulinic acid in the urine and increased free erythrocyte protoporphyrin (FEP). Lead causes partial inhibition of haem synthesis due to its effect on haem synthetase and δ-aminolaevulinic acid dehydratase. FEP is raised in iron deficiency but values above 500 μg/100 ml packed cells indicate lead toxicity.

Differential diagnoses of a space-occupying lesion and viral encephalitis are possible although the 6 months' history of behavioural changes makes the latter distinctly unlikely. Both generally present with headache and vomiting followed by localizing signs, not present in this case. Diminished reflexes with flexor plantars would be unlikely; upper motor neuron signs are more usual. A pyrexia occurs in lead poisoning either as a result of convulsions or from an intercurrent infection which can spark off the acute encephalopathy. Space-occupying lesions from whatever cause–abscess, subdural or tumour–may result in a temperature. Convulsions are fairly uncommon as a presentation of cerebral tumours in childhood, occurring in about 10% of patients. EEG and a CT scan would help in the diagnosis of these two conditions.

In view of the meningism present, meningitis must be considered. This could account for the acute illness, but with signs of raised intracranial pressure, a more chronic illness such as tuberculous meningitis (TBM) should come to mind. This would fit with the failure to thrive, but not with the other acute history. TBM usually has a history of about 2 weeks' drowsiness prior to coma and focal signs. The question of a lumbar puncture is a problem. It is very risky in view of the raised intracranial pressure and certainly the above conditions should be diagnosed by other less invasive techniques. In lead poisoning there is a mild pleocytosis and raised CSF protein value which will help very little in distinguishing it definitely from other conditions.

Lastly, in a comatose child who presents an unusual history (even if it is prolonged) that cannot be accounted for, drug intoxication should never be forgotten. This time it seems unlikely in view of the pyrexia and raised intracranial pressure.

Further reading

Braithwaite, R. A. and Brown, S. S. (1988). Clinical and sub-clinical lead poisoning: a laboratory perspective. *Human Toxicology*, **7**, 503–13.

Needleman, H. L. (1988). The persistent threat of lead: medical and sociological issues. *Current Problems in Pediatrics*, **18**, 697–744.

Veerula, G. R. and Noah, P. K. (1990). Clinical manifestations of childhood lead poisoning. *Journal of Tropical Medicine and Hygiene*, **93**, 170–7.

Case 6

Answers

1. (a) Abdominal ultrasound.
   (b) IVP with late films, i.e. 6 hours.
   (c) Repeat blood cultures.
   (d) Repeat urine cultures.
   (e) Technetium 99–DMSA renal scan.
2. Pyonephrosis/infected right hydronephrosis with ureteral obstruction.
3. (a) Drainage of pyonephrosis and nephrostomy.
   (b) Appropriate antibiotics for infecting organisms that will also cross the blood–brain barrier.

Discussion

A mass in the right side of the abdomen in a male baby could arise from kidney, liver, bowel, gallbladder or tumour. Throughout this boy's course in hospital he had no obvious bowel symptoms apart from vomiting, which could be accounted for by the urinary tract infection and meningitis; there was no palpable liver or jaundice. Instead he appeared to start with a urine infection, developed meningitis from the resulting septicaemia and then had a swinging temperature suggestive of a collection of pus. Subsequent urine microscopy and culture were negative. When this occurs in a child who appears to have continuing infection an obstructed kidney should be considered. To prove this may be difficult if no ultrasound is available. Intravenous urography should be done, but delayed films at about 6 hours or more are very useful. Sometimes the early films show only one kidney functioning. The same problem will occur in the DMSA renal scan. However, late films may show some contrast taken up on the obstructed side. Ultrasound has the added benefit that if the mass is not kidney, then its origin may be delineated.

Further urine cultures may not be helpful in this situation, but blood cultures may grow the organism. The antibiotics already employed will probably make culture difficult.

An obstructed infected kidney has to be relieved and the pus cultured. Since this child has definitely had partially treated meningitis, it is imperative that antibiotics used are appropriate

124

not only for the urinary tract infection but also cross the blood–brain barrier well. Examples are chloramphenicol, trimethoprim, cefotoxime and cefuroxime. Further treatment depends on the site of obstruction, its extent and whether it is extrinsic or intrinsic. In this child it was at the pelviureteric junction and required prolonged nephrostomy with a pelvoureteroplasty at a later date when the infection was cleared. It is important to try conservative surgery in a younger child and not perform a nephrectomy, since hydronephrosis is often bilateral with presentation at different ages.

Further reading

Edelmann, C. M. Jr. (ed.) (1978). *Pediatric Kidney Disease*, p. 1123. (Boston; Little, Brown)
Nixon, H. and O'Donnell, B. (1992). *Essentials of Paediatric Surgery*. 4th Edn. (Oxford; Butterworth-Heinemann)

Case 7

Answers

1. Anticonvulsant therapy.
2. Reduce, stop or change anticonvulsant therapy or add the daily requirement of vitamin D.

Discussion

The hypophosphataemia and elevated alkaline phosphatase activity suggest that this child has rickets. Collaborative evidence may be gained from X-rays of an epiphysis, and measurement of 25-hydroxycholecalciferol or parathormone. Aminoaciduria and occasionally glycosuria may be present but may be caused by renal damage in this patient. The two potential causes of rickets in this child are anticonvulsant therapy and renal damage; of these, anticonvulsant therapy is the more likely aetiological agent. Renal damage prevents the phosphaturic effect of parathormone causing hyperphosphataemia. Anticonvulsants, mainly phenobar-

bitone and phenytoin, cause vitamin D-deficient rickets by hepatic enzyme induction, producing an increased breakdown of
1,25-dihydroxycholecalciferol. The resultant hypocalcaemia induces secondary hyperparathyroidism which maintains serum
calcium at the expense of the skeletal pool. Parathormone has a
phosphaturic effect causing increased excretion of phosphate
and, therefore, hypophosphataemia.

Ideally, treatment would be to reduce, stop, or alter the anticonvulsant therapy; failing this, vitamin D supplements of 400 iu
daily should be given.

Further reading

Rall, T. W. and Schleifer, L. S. (1985). Drugs effective in the therapy of the
epilepsies. In *The Pharmacological Basis of Therapeutics*, 7th edn., Ed. by A. O.
Gilman, L. S. Goodman, T. W. Rall and F. Murad. pp. 446–72. (New York;
MacMillan)
Sinclair, L. (ed.) (1979). *Metabolic Disease in Childhood*, p. 181. (Oxford; Black-
well Scientific Publications)

Case 8

Answers

1. Subacute sclerosing panencephalitis (SSPE).
2. (a) Measles antibody titre.
   CSF measles antibody titre.
   EEG.

Discussion

SSPE usually presents between the ages of 5 and 15 years and is
associated with a raised blood and CSF IgG and IgM titres of
measles antibody. Clinical presentation is in 4 stages. The first
stage consists of insidious deterioration in behaviour and intellec-
tual performance plus small involuntary movements, occasional
falling backwards. The second stage is of increasing mental
deterioration with the involuntary jerky movements becoming
spasmodic and regular. Generalised restlessness, increasing

hypertonia, focal neurological deficits, falls, grand mal convulsions, cortical blindness and focal choroidorentinitis are seen. In the third stage there is increasing extra pyramidal and pyramidal dysfunction with rigidity and severe dementia, the patient becomes bedridden. Stage four is coma leading to death. EEG changes may be specific. The most distinctive feature is the occurrence of bilateral periodic complexes of high amplitude slow waves appearing usually every 5–7 s. These complexes coincide with a myoclonic jerk.

In an older child, the number of diseases causing regression is much fewer than in children under 18 months. Possible differential diagnoses in this child include: acute psychosis, minor motor seizures, Wilson's disease, Huntington's chorea or late-onset metachromatic leukodystrophy. Acute psychosis is unlikely in view of the slow onset but certainly may present with the clinical picture of acute encephalopathy. Both Wilson's disease and Huntington's chorea may present with dementia followed by extrapyramidal signs and choreiform movement in this age group. Younger children with Wilson's disease generally present with hepatic problems. Metachromatic leukodystrophy would be extremely unusual at the age of 12 years; presentation occurs around the age of 1 year with regression, ataxia and increasing spasticity. However, there is an adult form.

There are some very rare inborn errors of metabolism which should be considered when all the above have been excluded. These are:

1. Lafora body disease, a degenerative disease starting with epilepsy, then myoclonus and finally extrapyramidal signs, dementia and bulbar palsy.
2. Hallervorden–Spatz disease, in which pigmented material is deposited in the substantia nigra resulting in athetosis, rigidity and dementia.

Further reading

Bellman, M. H. and Dick, O. (1978). Sub-acute sclerosing panencephalitis. *Postgraduate Medical Journal*, **54**, 587-90.

Brett, E. M. (1991). *Paediatric Neurology*. Sub-acute Sclerosing Panencephalitis, pp. 633–8. (Edinburgh; Churchill Livingstone)

Neurologic Clinics (1985). *Paediatric Neurology. Sub-acute Sclerosing Panencephalitis: Current Status*, pp. 179–94

O'Donohoe, N. V. (1985). *Epilepsies of Childhood*. Post-graduate Paediatric Series, pp. 38–44, 114. (London; Butterworths)

Case 9

Answers

1. (a) Lumbar puncture.
   (b) Repeat blood culture.
   (c) Countercurrent immune electrophoresis.
   (d) Skeletal survey.
2. (a) Pneumococcal meningitis.
   (b) Osteomyelitis.
3. Penicillin G (benzyl penicillin) intravenously in high dose for 10–14 days.

Discussion

Pneumococcal infection is common in conjunction with sickle cell disease, particularly in the first years of life. The increased risk results from a deficiency of serum opsonins against pneumococci and the state of functional hyposplenism secondary to reduced phagocytic and reticuloendothelital functions. This is followed later by repeated episodes of infarction in the spleen. Any child with sickle cell disease whose temperature does not settle on what appears to be appropriate treatment for a specific infection, and who appears unwell, should be suspected of having pneumococcal meningitis or other infection. Approximately 10% of children with sickle cell disease develop pneumococcal sepsis or meningitis in the first 5 years of life. Pneumococcal meningitis has been reported as being 5–50 times more common in black children than white, and approximately 30 times more common in children with sickle cell disease than other black children.

Partially treated meningitis should be considered in the differential diagnosis of any child who remains unwell despite antibiotics, with signs of irritability or lethargy even in the absence of any meningism. Confirmation is obtained on lumbar puncture with an increased WBC count in the CSF, and raised protein, while culture is generally sterile. Countercurrent immunoelectrophoresis on CSF and blood with appropriate antiserum for pneumococci, meningococci and *Haemophilus influenzae* may help to identify the organism.

Treatment with penicillin in high dosage intravenously for at least 10 days is the treatment of choice. This is important because of the high mortality rate–approximately 25% in these cases.

A differential diagnosis in such a patient with sickle cell disease is osteomyelitis, possibly due to unusual organisms such as salmonella. This is unlikely in this case, first because the temperature appeared to respond to penicillin when given parenterally. Secondly, the patient did not have bone pain, which is generally an early sign and may follow a veno-occlusive crisis. Even if the pain is not localized there is usually reluctance to move the limb involved. Sickle cell crisis with abdominal pain is also a possibility and can be difficult to diagnose in a young child. Again there is usually pain and tenderness on palpation of the abdomen. The WBC is not usually helpful, since it is generally raised in sickle cell crisis with a neutrophilia, thus infection and crisis cannot be distinguished easily.

Further reading

Bell W. E. and McCormick W. F. (1975). *Neurologic Infections in Children. Pneumococcal Meningitis.* p. 180. (Philadelphia; Saunders)

Brett, E. M. (1991). *Paediatric Neurology.* Infections of the Nervous System, pp. 603–14. (Edinburgh; Churchill Livingstone)

Marshall, E. C. and Banforth, J. S. O. (1981). The impact of pneumococcal infections in paediatrics. In *Pneumonia and Pneumococcal Infections.* Royal Society of Medicine International Congress and Symposium Series, no. 27. (London; Royal Society of Medicine)

Serjeant, G. R. (1985). *Sickle Cell Disease. The Immune System*, pp. 124–34. (Oxford; Oxford University Press)

Case 10

Answers

1. Neuroblastoma in the cervical sympathetic chain.
2. (a) Urinary catecholamine metabolites.
   (b) Chest X-ray.
   (c) Marrow aspiration.
   (d) Angiography.
   (e) Alpha-fetoprotein.
   (f) Carcinoembryonic antigen.
   (g) Skeletal survey.

Discussion

The combination of gastroenterological symptoms and Horner's syndrome in a child is highly suggestive of a neuroblastoma. Either a primary lesion in the sympathetic chain or a secondary lesion in close proximity could disrupt the sympathetic outflow, causing Horner's syndrome; the chronic diarrhoea is caused by vasoactive intestinal peptide which is variably excreted by neuroblastomas. Hypokalaemia may be induced by persistent diarrhoea.

Diagnosis is confirmed by detecting increased levels of urinary catecholamine metabolites. Carcinoembryonic antigen and alphafetoprotein may be detected, usually in disseminated disease. Once the diagnosis has been established it is important to determine the extent of the disease, by such methods as ultrasound, bone scan, bone marrow aspiration and arteriography, as this will be a factor in determining treatment and prognosis.

Neuroblastoma is a relatively common tumour of young childhood, 40% occurring by 2 years, 90% by 10 years. It arises from neural crest cells, permitting a wide variety of clinical sites which is reflected in the protean clinical features and presentations. There may be anaemia from marrow infiltration, lymphadenopathy, hypertension, non-specific pain and symptoms such as pyrexia, malaise and vomiting. Bony metastases may present with bone pain and are particularly common in the skull, especially the orbit, causing raised intracranial pressure and ptosis. Deposits in proximity to the spinal column may cause stridor, urinary symptoms, or spinal cord and root compression if infiltration occurs.

Tumours occurring *in utero* may cause hypertension, headache and sweating in the mother. Many other presentations have been documented.

The prognosis depends on age, site, state and differentiation. Good prognostic factors include early staging and stage IVS, young presentation, primaries above the diaphragm and well-differentiated histology, although there are well-documented reports of poorly differentiated tumours spontaneously converting to ganglioneuromas.

The accepted staging is:

Stage I, confined to site of origin.
Stage II, extending beyond the original site but not across the midline.

Stage III, extending across the midline.

Stage IV, distant metastases.

Stage IVS, stage I and stage II with involvement of skin, muscle liver or bone marrow only.

Treatment for stages I and II is surgery while in stages III and IV chemotherapy followed by surgery is being tried. Stage IVS often remits spontaneously.

Further reading

Cheung, N. V. (1991). Immunotherapy: neuroblastoma as a model. *Pediatric Clinics of North America*, **38**, 425–41.

Kushner, B. H. and Cheung, N. K. (1988). Neuroblastoma. *Pediatric Annals*, **17**, 269–76, 278–84.

Nesbit, M. E. (1990). Advances and management of solid tumors in children. *Cancer*, **65** (suppl 3), 696–702.

Case 11

Answers

1. (a) Hypovolaemia.
   (b) Arterial thrombosis.
   (c) Peritonitis.
2. (a) Doppler of leg pulses.
   (b) Coagulation screen.
   (c) Aortogram.
   (d) Creatinine.
   (e) Blood culture.
3. (a) Insert central venous pressure (CVP) line.
   (b) Intravascular volume replacement followed by rehydration.
   (c) Steroids.
   (d) Anticoagulation.
   (e) Penicillin.

Discussion

Abdominal pain in nephrotic syndrome frequently heralds the onset of one of the major complications–hypovolaemia or peritonitis. Peritonitis was unlikely in view of the prolonged history, lack of temperature when off steroids and lack of increasing abdominal signs. Hypovolaemia, on the other hand, was very likely right from the start. It often presents with abdominal pain and vomiting and these, compounded with postural hypotension and cool peripheries, are almost conclusive. However, it is easy to make a diagnosis of relapsed nephrotic syndrome secondary to infective gastroenteritis and feel that things will sort themselves out, but fluid balance in an already hypovolaemic patient should be very carefully watched. Following her progress further, weight loss after admission in a patient with nephrotic syndrome and heavy proteinuria is unusual. The dehydration is depicted by the rise in Hb and possibly urea, although the lack of creatinine level makes it impossible to say whether renal function is compromised.

If a patient is thought to have severe hypovolaemia he or she should be treated with salt-poor albumin, 0.5–1 g/kg given cautiously depending on serum albumin and, if necessary, plasma infusion. Following volume replacement, which can be judged on CVP, rehydration should be started according to the biochemistry.

The second problem this child presents with is ischaemia of the lower limbs. Initially she could be thought to have just poor perfusion, but the history is typical of an ischaemic limb, i.e. cool temperature, pain and tenderness progressing to lack of sensation, and then lack of movement. A hypercoagulability state has frequently been described in nephrotic syndrome–reports of arterial thromboses, femoral vein thromboses after venepuncture and the endless argument as to whether renal vein thrombosis is cause or effect of nephrotic syndrome. In view of the above history a clotting screen should be carried out, Doppler soundings of the pulses obtained, especially after volume replacement, and if there is no improvement then the patient should be anticoagulated–some success has been reported with streptokinase–and an aortogram carried out. In general if thrombosis has occurred, the relevant arteriogram or venogram should be done.

As far as further treatment is concerned, penicillin can be added as a prophylactic against pneumococcal infection after a

132

blood culture and the relapse should be treated with steroids, initially intravenously.

Further reading

Baker, M. R. (1979). Two cases of nephrotic syndrome with reversible coagulation defect. *Postgraduate Medical Journal*, **55**, 648, 757–61.

Egan, T. J. *et al.* (1967). Shock as a complication of nephrotic syndrome. *American Journal of Diseases in Childhood*, **113**, 364.

Grupe, W. E. (1986). Management of primary nephrotic syndrome. In *Clinical Paediatric Nephrology*, Ed. by Postlethwaite R. J., pp. 175–96. (Bristol; Wright)

Kendall, A. G., Lohmann, R. C. and Dossetor, J. B. (1971). Nephrotic syndrome; a hyper-coagulability state. *Archives of Internal Medicine*, **127**, 1021

Vahaskari, V. M. (1981). The nephrotic syndrome in children. *Pediatric Annals*, **10**, 42–64.

Case 12

Answers

1. Somogyi effect.
2. (a) 24-hour fractional urine collections.
   (b) Blood sugar profile.
   (c) 12-hour fractional urinary free cortisols.
3. (a) Lower the insulin dose.
   (b) Change insulin to one with a different time action, a biphasic insulin e.g. 30% fast-acting/70% Isophane, or a twice-daily regime.

Discussion

A child whose diabetic control is good, as shown by low glycosuria and glycolysated Hb, who also has episodes of ketosis and hyperglycosuria, is probably manifesting the Somogyi effect. This is a phenomenon where hypoglycaemia is followed rapidly by hyperglycaemia as a result of the body over-reacting to the fall in blood sugar. Some children show little or nothing in the way of clinical signs to hypoglycaemia. Night-time hypoglycaemia can be a worry to many parents of diabetic children, and may be very difficult to prove. It can be easy to raise the insulin dose in the face of proven glycosuria. An escalating insulin dose may result as described here. Any insulin with a fast-acting component may produce the Somogyi effect towards the end of the morning, but this child is on a long-acting insulin and one should be aware that glycosuria and ketosis do not always indicate poor control.

Improved control should result if the insulin dose is reduced, or divided and given twice daily. Alternatively a change to a biphasic insulin or one with a different duration of action may be tried. Changing the diet to give a heavy carbohydrate load at night is not a satisfactory course of action.

The simplest test to try to demonstrate a Somogyi effect is a 24-hour fractional urine test. Urine is collected in four timed intervals. In this child glycosuria should be low during the day but the overnight specimen from 8 p.m. to 8 a.m. should show much heavier glycosuria. This will only suggest but not prove the diagnosis. Home blood glucose monitoring is now routine and could be very helpful here, but would require night-time samples. Urinary free cortisols are a method of assessing the 'stress' caused by an unrecognized episode of hypoglycaemia. Careful timing of the samples may show unexpectedly high urinary cortisols at night.

Further reading

Craig, O. (1981). *Childhood Diabetes and its Management*, 2nd edn. Postgraduate Paediatric Series. (London; Butterworths)

Kinmonth, A. L. and Baum, J. D. (1984). Dietary management of diabetes. In *Recent Advances in Paediatrics* no. 7 Ed. by Meadow R., pp. 197–215. (London; Churchill Livingstone).

Case 13

Answers

1. (a) Blood pressure.
   (b) Palpable gonads.

   (c) Pigmentation.
2. (a) Congenital adrenal hyperplasia (CAH).
   (b) Salt-losing crisis.
3. (a) Plasma 17-hydroxyprogesterone.
   (b) Renin.
   (c) Aldosterone.
   (d) Androstenedione.

Discussion

This child has ambiguous genitalia; the most important diagnosis to exclude, therefore, is CAH as a number of these infants suffer from salt-losing crisis. Pigmentation of the infant would suggest CAH, via increased melanocyte stimulating hormone (MSH) activity secondary either to release of MSH from the pars intermedia of the pituitary, or cross-reaction with adrenocorticotrophic hormone (ACTH). CAH is recessively inherited; it is, therefore, probable that the sibling died from a salt-losing crisis rather than 'gastroenteritis'. Hypertension in the infant would suggest a 17-hydroxylase deficiency in which salt-losing crises do not occur. The commonest enzyme deficiency causing ambiguous genitalia with salt-losing crisis is 21-hydroxylase deficiency. 3-Hydroxysteroid dehydrogenase deficiency may produce a similar situation, but is far less common. The crisis usually occurs during the first 3 weeks of life, so fluid and electrolyte balance must be carefully monitored in the neonatal period. Diagnosis is made by determining excess precursors prior to 21 hydroxylation, such as plasma 17-hydroxyprogesterone. However, this metabolite is normally high during the first 48 hours, especially in the preterm child and in infants stressed by infection or surgery. Renin and aldosterone estimation may be helpful in elucidating the problem.

Only a percentage of infants with 21-hydroxylase deficiency suffer salt-losing crisis, although the enzyme is part of the mineralocorticoid pathway. The reason is unknown; isoenzymes and second gene loci have been postulated. Individual enzyme deficiencies are elucidated by detailed analysis of precursors and metabolites. Life-long treatment with mineralo- and glucocorticoids is indicated.

Palpable gonads are virtually always testes; ovaries rarely migrate outside the pelvis. If gonads are palpable in an apparent female, CAH is a tenable diagnosis. The enzyme deficiency would be 20,22-desmolase or 3-hydroxysteroid dehydrogenase deficiency, both resulting in a salt-losing crisis, or 17,20-desmolase deficiency, not associated with dehydration.

Once CAH has been excluded the diagnosis requires further investigative procedures. Chromosome analysis affords genetic sex; . phenotypic sex is judged on both internal and external genitalia, usually localized by radiography.

In males there may be a defect in androgen production either peripherally or, rarely, secondary to hypopituitarism. End-organ unresponsiveness to testosterone–testicular feminization syndrome–results in normal female genitalia in the presence of normal circulating testosterone values.

Female virilization is commonly secondary to CAH; other causes include maternal drugs or virilizing tumour during pregnancy, or idiopathic virilization.

The sexual and psychological management of these children is determined by the best function afforded by the external genitalia.

Further reading

New, M. I. and Speiser, P. W. (1989). Congenital adrenal hyperplasia. In *Clinical Paediatric Endocrinology*, 2nd edn. Ed. by C. G. D. Brook. (Oxford; Blackwell Scientific Publications)

Pagon, R. A. (1987). Diagnostic approach to the newborn with ambiguous genitalia. *Pediatric Clinics of North America*, **34**, 1019–31.

Tindall, V. R. (1987). Sex determination, asexuality and intersexuality. In *Jeffcoate's Principles of Gynaecology*, 5th edn, Ed. by V. R. Tindall, pp. 159–84. (London; Butterworths)

Case 14

Answers

1. A toxicological screen of blood and urine.

Discussion

This child was admitted four times before her death with bizarre, unexplained neurological signs and symptoms. At each admission the signs resolved rapidly without treatment or neurological sequelae. In these circumstances drug-induced illness must be excluded by a toxicological screen for the more common psychotropic drugs. In this case, it may have saved the child's life. Children are notoriously adept at acquiring 'safe' drugs; helpful and more ingenious siblings may also be a source of danger.

The mother was reported as suffering from postpartum depression. Contact with her general practitioner revealed that she had been referred to a psychiatrist, who had prescribed imipramine.

Under further questioning mother admitted deliberately giving the child imipramine as she had felt unable to cope with both children.

Analysis of the stomach contents and blood postmortem revealed high levels of imipramine and desipramine, the metabolite. Signs that should have alerted the practitioner were hypotension and tachycardia, especially supraventricular tachycardia. ECG changes are non-specific, but there may be flattening or inversion of the T wave. Other features include mydriasis and sluggish reflexes, dry mouth and flushed dry skin, hypothermia, blurred vision and urinary retention. Apnoea occurs only with high toxic blood levels.

Non-accidental poisoning of children is being reported with increasing incidence, as also is Münchausen's syndrome by proxy, possibly a related phenomenon. Often one or other of the parents has a psychiatric history and may have some medical knowledge. Various hypotheses, including marital disharmony, have been postulated for this form of child abuse but none substantiated.

Treatment requires long-term psychiatric care of the family, or in extreme cases removal of the child.

Further reading

Barkin, R. M. (1990). Toxicologic emergencies. *Pediatric Annals* **19**, 629–33.

Craft, A. W. (1983). Circumstances surrounding deaths from accidental poisoning. 1974–80. *Archives of Disease in Childhood*, **58**, 544–6.

Meadow, R. (1977). Münchausen syndrome by proxy. The hinterland of child abuse. *Lancet*, **ii**, 343.

Mehl, A. L. (1990). Münchausen syndrome by proxy: a family affair. *Child Abuse and Neglect*, **14**, 577–85.

Case 15

Answers

1. (a) Postictal state.
   (b) Fresh-water drowning.
   (c) Subarachnoid haemorrhage.
   (d) Drug intoxication/poisoning.
   (e) Subdural haemorrhage.
2. (a) Repeat electrolytes.
   (b) Blood gases.
   (c) Drug screen.
   (d) CT scan.
   (e) Lumbar puncture.
   (f) EEG.

Discussion

In view of the poor history it is difficult to make any diagnosis with certainty. A serious head injury is unlikely with no skull fracture, as is subdural haematoma since there was no lucid interval. Spontaneous cerebral insult such as a bleeding arteriovenous malformation, arterial embolus or thrombus is a possibility, but no focal CNS signs make this less likely. Subarachnoid haemorrhage should result in neck stiffness and subhyaloid haemorrhages in the eye, but there are always exceptions, and this should be excluded by CT scan or lumbar puncture.

Metabolic problems in a child who has been well right up to the period of unconsciousness would appear to be a remote possibility; the blood glucose value is normal. However, there are abnormalities of the electrolytes. These at first glance could represent fresh-water drowning, but on closer examination this seems unlikely. Survivors who arrive for treatment after an episode of near drowning will manifest only transient electrolyte changes, which will revert to normal without specific fluid and electrolyte therapy. In one study (Modell *et al.*) victims of fresh-water aspiration had a mean serum sodium level of 138 mmol/litre and serum potassium level of 3.9 mmol/litre. The ranges regardless of sea- or fresh-water aspiration were: sodium, 126–160 mmol/litre; and potassium, 2.4–6.3 mmol/litre.

Most victims die from other factors, probably anoxia and acidosis. Aspiration of as little as 2.2 ml/kg of water in animals produces profound changes in Pa_{O_2}, which can be accounted for by a large intrapulmonary shunt with a ventilation–perfusion imbalance. Fresh water is absorbed from the alveoli but causes alteration of pulmonary surfactant followed by atelectasis. Hypoxia continues into the recovery phase for a period of 72 hours or more. PaC_{O_2} may rise initially but rapidly returns to normal when the patient hyperventilates. A metabolic acidosis is also persistent and marked, probably due to tissue hypoxia. Thus blood gases could be a valuable investigation. Hb and haematocrit are usually in normal ranges in near-drowning victims; haemolysis does occur but is seldom of such a degree to necessitate specific therapy. None of the above features are present in the patient described: cyanosis was short-lived and the blood film was normal, thus is seems possible that the low sodium level was erroneous, either through laboratory error or blood taken through an intravenous line; it should be repeated.

This boy could be in a postictal state. However, there is no convincing history, and the fact that he swam to the side of the pool suggests a short-lived episode which would not generally be followed by a prolonged period of drowsiness. The momentary shaking and cyanosis at the pool-side and on admission could be shivering. An EEG is the simplest investigation, if available, and should show an epileptic focus, although this may be difficult to differentiate from an abnormal wave pattern secondary to cerebral abnormality or insult. Since CT scans are now widely available, this has become one of the first-line investigations for any patient who has a period of depressed consciousness of unknown aetiology, and is safer than a lumbar puncture.

In fact the diagnosis was self-poisoning and was first suspected from the EEG which showed signs of drug toxicity. On regaining consciousness he admitted to taking his mother's Valium (diazepam) and barbiturate sleeping tablets in the lunch hour. This underlines the necessity of always taking blood and urine for a drug screen when a child presents in unusual circumstances, especially when one family member is depressed or known to be on medication, or if the family relationships are unusual. Poisoning may be deliberate on the part of patient or parent.

Further reading

Aicardi, J. (1985). Epileptic syndromes in childhood. In *Paediatric Perspectives on Epilepsy*, Ed. by E. Ross and E. Reynolds, pp. 65–71. (Chichester; J. Wiley)

Eeg-Olofsson, O. (1985). Types of epilepsy in the young schoolchild. In *Paediatric Perspectives on Epilepsy*, Ed. by E. Ross and E. Reynolds, pp. 103–10. (Chichester; J. Wiley)

Meadow, R. (1984). Factitious illness: the hinterland of child abuse. *Recent Advances in Paediatrics*, **7**, 217–31.

Modell, J. H., Graves, S. A. and Ketover, A. (1976). Clinical course of 91 consecutive near drowning victims. *Chest*, **70**, 231.

O'Donohoe, N. (1985). Major generalized epilepsy and partial seizures of complex symptomatology. In *Epilepsies of Childhood*, Postgraduate Paediatrics Series, pp. 76–81; 92–104 (London; Butterworths)

Case 16

Answers

1. (a) Erythema multiforme.
   (b) Stevens–Johnson syndrome.
2. (a) *Myoplasma pneumoniae* infection.
   (b) Viral, particularly herpes simplex.
   (c) Bacterial infection, e.g. typhoid, focal sepsis.
   (d) Drug sensitivity, particularly sulphonamides and penicillin.
   (e) Infectious mononucleosis.
   (f) Collagen diseases, e.g. systemic lupus erythematosus (SLE).
3. (a) Attack subsides over 2–3 weeks, giving full recovery.

Discussion

This child presents a classic picture of erythema multiforme, which may be precipitated by a wide variety of factors, such as viral infections especially herpes simplex, mycoplasma, bacterial infections, histoplasmosis and almost any drug. There are three main clinical varieties. First, the papular form which is the commonest, involving hands, feet and extensor surfaces of the limbs. The lesions consist of heliotrope papules and plaques of variable diameter up to 2 cm. Central discoloration of these plaques produces the characteristic target lesion. Secondly, the vesico-bullous form of skin lesions in which the oral mucosa is also involved. Thirdly, the Stevens–Johnson syndrome, which is a very severe form of bullous erythema multiforme in which the eyes, mouth and genitalia may also be involved. Two such mucous membranes should be involved to make this diagnosis. There is also a severe systemic upset with fever, polyarthritis, diarrhoea or pneumonia. Conjunctivitis and photophobia may be marked.

Although this child does not fit neatly into one of these classic varieties, he probably is nearest to the Stevens–Johnson form because of the mouth and eye involvement, together with the severe systemic upset. A very important differential diagnosis is Kawasaki disease. The clinical features of this disease may include fever; a generalized, often urticarial or morbilliform rash, then desquamation of the palms and soles, fingers and toes; lymphadenopathy; conjunctival injection; pharyngitis; cracking of the lips; 'strawberry' tongue; arthritis and jaundice. There is a neutrophil leukocytosis, a sterile pyuria and a thrombocytosis. Cardiac complications, i.e. myocarditis and coronary artery aneurysms, occur in 20–40% of patients, causing 1–2% mortality. The aetiology of this disease is unknown. Viral infections, e.g. echo- and adenovirus may give rise to a similar combination of symptoms and signs but usually not as florid. Other differential diagnoses include urticaria, toxic erythema, erythema nodosum–but the lesions are not typical–and dermatitis herpetiformis which is rare in childhood, particularly at this age; the rash has a different distribution and is very itchy.

The aetiology in this child was never found as in 50% of such cases, despite there being some features of bacterial infection, i.e. polymorph leukocytosis and low CSF sugar values. He probably had a viral infection; there was no history of drug ingestion.

Treatment is supportive, and any specific infection is treated appropriately. Offending drugs should be withdrawn, and Stevens–Johnson syndrome may be treated with systemic corti-costeroids, but this is controversial. The attack gradually subsides over 2–3 weeks with complete recovery, but recurrent episodes may occur.

Further reading

Cassidy, J. R. and Petty, R. E. (1990). *Textbook of Pediatric Rheumatology*, pp. 385–94. (New York; Churchill Livingstone)

Cuttica, R. J. (1990). Kawasaki disease and vasculopathies. *Current Opinion in Rheumatology*, **2**, 809–16.

Harper, J. (1990). *Handbook of Paediatric Dermatology*, pp. 87–92. (Oxford; Butterworth-Heinemann)

Taaffe, A. G. (1975). The Stevens–Johnson syndrome. *British Journal of Clinical Practice*, **29**, 169–71.

Case 17

Answers

1. (a) Malrotation with intermittent volvulus.
   (b) Duplication cyst of the upper small bowel.
2. Contrast studies of the bowel.

Discussion

There are numerous causes of childhood vomiting, both surgical and medical; however, the abdominal X-ray suggests a surgical cause. The stomach and duodenum were dilated with reabsorption of gas from the distal gut, implying an obstruction in the duodenum or proximal jejunum. This is supported by the vomiting being forceful and bile-stained, and also by the metabolic alkalosis.

The recurrent nature of the attacks, without diarrhoea, suggests an intermittent, spontaneously resolving obstruction. Intermittent volvulus secondary to malrotation is, therefore, the most likely diagnosis. Volvulus secondary to a duplication cyst is a rarer possibility. Volvulus without malrotation is also rare and virtually always presents in the neonatal period. Confirmation can be gained by contrast studies using either air or a water-soluble medium, rather than barium, as infarction with subsequent perforation is a potential complication.

The commonest type of malrotation is limited rotation of the bowel through 180° only, resulting in the superior mesenteric artery and caecum lying anterior to the duodenum. Connections from the caecal visceral peritoneum to the parietal peritoneum in the right hypochondrium (Ladd's bands) may obstruct the second part of the duodenum, or the gut may rotate around the superior mesenteric artery. Less commonly, the initial 90° rotation of the gut occurs, the duodenum lying anterior to the superior mesenteric artery but, thereafter, variable degrees of rotation or non-rotation occur. Volvulus occurs around the short pedicle of small bowel mesentery. Rarer causes still are congenital kinks or bends or the bowel spiralling on itself.

Duplication cysts can be either tubular, running some length of the bowel, or small cysts. Obstruction is caused by the gut being stretched over a dilated cyst or by the heavier double bowel rotating around the mesentery. Duplication cysts of the duodenum are rare, but those of the small bowel are more common. If there is communication between the bowel lumen and duplication cyst, bacterial overgrowth may occur with the subsequent blind loop syndrome.

Treatment for these conditions is surgical.

Further reading

Bill, A. H. (1980). Malrotation and failures of fixation of the intestinal tract. In *Pediatric Surgery*, Ed. by T. M. Holder and K. W. Ashcroft, pp. 346–55. (Philadelphia; W. B. Saunders)

Black, J. A. (ed.) (1987). Medical conditions which may mimic an acute abdominal emergency. In *Paediatric Emergencies*, 2nd edn. Postgraduate Paediatrics Series, pp. 375–90. (London; Butterworths)

Lister, J. (1990). Duplication of the alimentary tract. In *Neonatal Surgery*, 3rd edn. Ed. by J. Lister and I. M. Irving, pp. 474–83. (London; Butterworths)

Case 18

Answers

1. (a) Vascular incident, particularly arterial occlusion or bleed from a vascular malformation.
   (b) Idiopathic.
   (c) Encephalitis.
   (d) Postictal.
2. (a) CT scan.
   (b) Skull X-rays.
   (c) ECG.
   (d) Chest X-ray.
   (e) Echocardiography.

Discussion

Acute hemiplegia in a young child is not rare and can occur secondary to a surprising variety of pathologies. There appear to be very few rules that help point to a specific aetiology. There are both vascular and non-vascular causes: viral and bacterial infections, trauma, immunizations, systemic disease, arteriovenous malformations, cardiac abnormalities, status epilepticus and neoplasms are just some examples.

The classic description was given by Freud of a previously healthy child who suddenly becomes ill from the age of a few months to 3 years. The initial symptoms may be violent–with fever, convulsions and vomiting–or may be slight or insignificant. Infantile hemiplegia is not a disease, but rather a non-specific response of the CNS to multiple and varied conditions. In a significant number of cases, varying in different series, no specific aetiology is found. Isler (1971), pre CT scan, has probably provided the most comprehensive series of 116 cases in which the causes were as follows: arterial occlusions (31); vascular malformations (21); cerebral diseases, i.e. postictal and encephalitis (46); migraine accompagnee (9); the remainder were venous occlusions and subdural haematomata.

Onset may also be intermittent or 'stuttering', as in this case, and is classic of thrombosis, although this is unreliable. This child had spontaneous occlusion of the left middle cerebral artery for no apparent reason. This can, of course, occur secondary to another disease process such as sickle cell disease or SLE. The middle cerebral artery is also the usual site for emboli which may come from the heart secondary to infective endocarditis and cardiac arrhythmias, or from a lesion in the lungs. Hence the necessity for cardiological investigations with chest X-ray, ECG, and possibly echocardiogram, even without a clinical pointer to a cardiological problem.

Cerebral haemorrhage can present in varied fashion; children with haematological problems such as leukaemia, thrombocytopenic purpura and sickle cell disease are particularly at risk. Blood usually leaks into the subarachnoid space, causing neck stiffness. Subarachnoid haemorrhage itself is generally secondary to vascular malformations, such as arteriovenous malformations, angiomas and aneurysms. A carotid angiogram used to be necessary for diagnosis of these abnormalities since they may not show up on a CT scan. Carotid angiography in the acute phase is not dangerous in experienced hands, but with the advent of the MRI scanner, this would be the preferred investigation. Hypertension should never be forgotten as a cause of cerebral haemorrhage, even in a child.

Encephalitis is occasionally complicated by hemiplegia but in the early stages may be focal and cause a vasculitis. Herpes simplex is the best-documented viral cause of focal encephalitis and should be excluded by CT scan, if available, since it causes necrotic areas, particularly in the temporal lobe. Since this is a treatable cause, acyclovir should be started while awaiting results of investigations. Other viruses such as enteroviruses, mumps, measles and influenza have been implicated, as has immunization with pertussis, measles, rubella and recently the measles, mumps and rubella (MMR) vaccine. The EEG may be helpful but sometimes is non-specific with discharges on the contralateral side to the brain lesion which could be explained by cerebral oedema or ischaemia. The CSF findings in this case would support a viral encephalitis but are not diagnostic and viral screen is negative.

In cases of hemiplegia it is imperative that conditions requiring specific treatment are diagnosed. These include space-occupying lesions–particularly subdural haematoma, brain abscess and tumours–bacterial meningitis and any underlying pathology such as pulmonary sepsis. Subdural haematoma often result from mild injury, but in about 50% of cases there is no history of trauma and no radiographic evidence of a fracture, thus skull X-rays are not always helpful. Features against it in this child are the fairly sudden onset and lack of signs of raised intracranial pressure. Cerebral abscess is also unlikely in view of the sudden onset, lack of pyrexia and site of origin of infection, and the CSF findings. Cerebral tumours are generally infratentorial in children presenting with signs of raised intracranial pressure and cerebellar involvement. Hemiplegic migraine is not usually a problem in this age group, generally not starting before puberty. The absence of headache and family history is also against the diagnosis. Migraine should always be kept in mind in a patient with sudden onset, then resolution of hemiplegia.

Further reading

Brett, E. M. (1991). *Paediatric Neurology*. Acute Hemiplegia, pp. 553–5. (Edinburgh; Churchill Livingstone)

Golden, G. S. (1985). *Stroke Syndromes in Childhood*. Neurological Clinics *(vol. 3:1)*: Paediatric Neurology, pp. 59–75 (Philadelphia; Saunders)

Isler, W. (1971). *Acute Hemiplegias and Hemisyndromes in Childhood*. (London; Heinemann)

Case 19

Answers

1. (a) Acute leukaemia–usually lymphoblastic (ALL) but could be myeloblastic (AML).
   (b) Aplastic anaemia.
   (c) Juvenile chronic arthritis (JCA).
   (d) Lymphoma–non-Hodgkin's.
   (e) Human immunodeficiency virus (HIV) infection.
2. (a) Bone marrow aspiration/trephine biopsy.
   (b) Leukaemic markers–immunological and enzymatic.
   (c) Bone marrow cytogenetics.
   (d) Lymph node biopsy.
   (e) Autoantibodies including DNA autoantibodies, and rheumatoid factor.
   (f) Blood culture.
   (g) Skeletal survey (or technetium bone scan).
   (h) Viral studies, including screen of pharyngeal washings, urine, stool and blood.
   (i) Hepatitis B serology.
   (j) HIV antibodies.

Discussion

The main diagnoses here are ALL and aplastic anaemia. Both these diseases usually present with symptoms and signs of anaemia, thrombocytopenia or neutropenia, i.e. lethargy, malaise, bleeding and infection. In aplastic anaemia there is no organomegaly as is present in this case, making aplasia unlikely. One of the main differences is that leukaemia can present with bone pain due to leukaemic infiltration. A viral infection preceding the onset of aplastic anaemia may produce limb pains, but these should have disappeared prior to the onset of symptoms of aplasia, which should occur 4–6 weeks later. Skeletal survey may reveal periosteal reaction and lytic lesions, which do not necessarily correlate with the sites of bone pain. These do not occur in aplastic anaemia. A technetium-99 scan could also be done to demonstrate skeletal 'hot spots', i.e. involvement.

When ALL presents with aplasia, bone marrow aspiration is unlikely to yield enough cells to allow any differentiation from aplastic anaemia to be made. A trephine biopsy is mandatory and hopefully a diagnosis can be made. Blood and marrow should be sent for leukaemic markers which are immunological (four types: T, B, common, null); cytogenetic markers which are important in predicting outcome (polyploidy is associated with good prognosis); and enzymatic markers, for example, terminal transferase, which is positive in common and T-cell ALL.

Lymph node biopsy may be helpful, especially if lymphadenopathy is marked. Cervical lymphadenopathy, as noted in this case, is common in the presentation of lymphoma, both Hodgkin's and non-Hodgkin's. Bone marrow involvement does occur, but aplasia is unlikely to be the main presentation. Usual signs are more localized lymphadenopathy, mediastinal masses which can be symptomatic with progressive dyspnoea, or palpable abdominal masses. Bone involvement may occur with resulting pain.

About 50% of cases of aplastic anaemia can be attributed to viral infections, chemicals or drugs. Of particular note is hepatitis B infection, thus hepatitis B serology is important. Immunological factors may also be important, therefore autoantibodies are relevant, as they are in JCA.

ALL mimics JCA if bone and joint pains predominate. Systemic JCA (Still's disease) with generalized lymphadenopathy, fever, abdominal pain, splenomegaly, together with the raised ESR, is also similar, but in this case there was no rash during the fever, which occurs in the majority of patients. Aplasia does not occur as a complication and obviously one should be wary of making a diagnosis of JCA in such a case without first ruling out leukaemia.

Infection often complicates the presentation and treatment of ALL, therefore a blood culture must be done. This little girl not only had numerous lytic lesions but also osteomyelitis of the leg.

Finally congenital HIV infection could present in a 2-year-old, particularly if the parents fall into any of the 'high-risk' categories.

Further reading

Cassidy, J. T. and Petty, R. E. (1990). *Textbook and Paediatric Rheumatology*, pp. 113–200. (New York; Churchill Livingstone)

Civin, L. I. and Pochedly, C. (eds) *Haematology/Oncology Clinics of North America* (August and October 1990), Childhood Acute Lymphoblastic Leukaemia. Parts 1 (vol. 4:4) and 2 (vol. 4:5). (Philadelphia; Saunders)

Gordon-Smith, E. C. (1989). *Aplastic Anaemia. Clinical Haematology–International Practice and Research*. (London; Baillière Tindall)

McElwain, T. I. (1979). Hodgkin's disease. In *Topics in Paediatrics. I. Haematology and Oncology*, Ed. by P. H. Morris-Jones, p. 84. (London; Pitman)

Case 20

Answers

1. (a) Hypoglycaemia.
   (b) Infection.
   (c) Apnoea of prematurity.
   (d) Intraventricular haemorrhage.
2. (a) Blood glucose or screening stix test.
   (b) Blood culture/bacterial swabs.
   (c) Lumbar puncture.
   (d) Chest X-ray.
   (e) Viral IgM antibodies.
   (f) High vaginal swab from mother.
3. Apnoea of prematurity.
4. (a) Continuous positive airways pressure.
   (b) Xanthine derivatives.

Discussion

This infant was premature and also small for dates, the birth weight being below the 10th centile, probably secondary to his mother's smoking habits. Both these factors result in reduced hepatic glycogen deposition, rendering the infant susceptible to hypoglycaemia which may occur in the first 24 hours of life. This must be excluded by Dextrostix with a confirmatory blood glucose estimation.

Asymptomatic hypoglycaemia has a good prognosis for future neurological development; however, symptomatic hypoglycaemia, implying severe cerebral hypoglycaemia, carries a poor prognosis with up to 60% of infants having neurological sequelae. Treatment of asymptomatic hypoglycaemia is with increased intake of oral glucose; symptomatic hypoglycaemia requires prompt intravenous therapy.

Infection is always a hazard in the neonatal period, especially in the premature baby, whose immune responses are immature. This infant was born after prolonged rupture of membranes, increasing the possibility of infection. Signs of infection include lethargy, poor feeding, apnoeic episodes and convulsions. The temperature may be unstable and the WBC is not helpful in the first 48 hours, varying in a non-specific way. Therefore, other investigations, such as blood culture, lumbar punctures, bacterial swabs and viral titres must be undertaken. This mother did not attend an antenatal clinic so nothing is known of her viral status.

The infant may have congenital pneumonia from infected liquor or an ascending infection, from the mother's vaginal and perineal flora. A chest X-ray may show patchy shadowing or lobar consolidation as opposed to the diffuse 'ground-glass' appearance of respiratory distress syndrome. Group B haemolytic streptococcus is prevalent in the UK with up to 41% of pregnant women colonized. It inhabits the cervix, the infant becoming infected during parturition. A septicaemia results, often with accompanying meningitis and pneumonia. The signs may mimic respiratory distress syndrome; differentiation is made by X-ray. A high vaginal swab from the mother may reveal the presence of the streptococcus.

Various investigations have been suggested as useful in the early detection of neonatal sepsis. These include ESR, total WBC, acute-phase proteins and gastric washings for WBC in prolonged rupture of membranes. All these investigations have too high a false-negative rate to be used definitively. The decision to start antibiotic therapy is often clinical.

Intraventricular haemorrhages have been detected in a high percentage of premature infants. The infants do not always have previous pathology, but predisposing factors include prematurity, hypoxia, hypercapnoea and positive pressure ventilation. The symptoms depend on the extent of the haemorrhage; a small intracerebral bleed may be manifest by poor feeding, irritability and apnoea, whereas a major bleed is often fatal. Diagnosis is by ultrasound or CT scan. Although this child had recurrent apnoeic attacks, the history states that the infant was otherwise well, which is against all but the most minor of intraventricular haemorrhages.

Idiopathic respiratory distress syndrome may occur in an infant of 33 weeks' gestation; however, there are usually early signs of respiratory embarrassment within the first 4 hours after birth, such as grunting, subcostal recession and flaring of the alae nasi. It is unusual for recurrent apnoea to be the presenting sign of respiratory distress syndrome.

No abnormalities were detected on initial examination, during investigations or subsequently; the most likely diagnosis is, therefore, apnoea of prematurity. The periods of apnoea are short and not accompanied by bradycardia and acidosis; however, it is a diagnosis of exclusion and other causes should be sought.

The infant should be placed on an apnoea alarm mattress and

can be stimulated at each apnoeic episode. Alternatively, the infant may be treated with xanthine derivatives, such as aminophylline or caffeine, or with continuous positive airways pressure.

Further reading

Baker, C. J. and Edwards, M. S. (1990). Group B streptococcal infections. In *Infectious Diseases of the Fetus and Newborn Infant*, 3rd edn, Ed. by J. S. Remington and J. O. Klein, pp. 742–811. (Philadelphia; W. B. Saunders)

Brown, J. K. and Minns, R. A. (1988). Apnoeic attacks. In *Fetal and Neonatal Neurology and Neurosurgery*, Ed. by M. I. Levene, M. J. Bennett and J. Punt, pp. 492–3. (London; Churchill Livingstone)

Miller, J. M. (1990). Strategies to prevent group B streptococcal neonatal sepsis. *Infections in Medicine*, 18–32

Wigglesworth, J. S. (1984). Perinatal infection. In *Perinatal Pathology*, Ed. by J. L. Bennington, pp. 159–60. (Philadelphia; W. B. Saunders)

Wigglesworth, J. S. (1984). The central nervous system. In *Perinatal Pathology*, Ed. by J. L. Bennington, pp. 263–71. (Philadelphia; W. B. Saunders)

Case 21

Answers

1. Approximately in the region of T3–4–anterior pressure on cord.
2. Chronic granulomatous disease (CGD).
3. (a) Spinal X-ray.
   (b) MRI scan, but myelogram if unavailable.
   (c) Nitroblue tetrazolium (NBT) test.
   (d) Tests for neutrophil function, i.e. chemotaxis, adhesion, phagocytosis, oxidation and bacterial killing.
   (e) Aspergillus precipitins.
   (f) Exclusion of tuberculosis with Mantoux and if necessary, bronchoscopy.
4. (a) Spinal decompression.
   (b) Amphotericin/antifungal agent.
   (c) White cell transfusion.
   (d) Physiotherapy.

Discussion

A 'cold' abscess on the chest wall, chest symptoms and signs, together with paraplegia, strongly suggest a diagnosis of tuberculosis. However, aspergillus was grown from the abscess fluid. This could have been a contaminant, but has shown to be pathogenic in several clinical situations recently, for example, asthma, cystic fibrosis and the immunocompromised. The presence of aspergillus precipitins will confirm that it is pathogenic and not a contaminant.

This child presents with a history dating back to the age of 5 months of recurrent infections including bronchitis, cervical lymphadenitis and perianal abscess, together with failure to thrive and hepatosplenomegaly. This is a classic presentation of CGD, which may also cause osteomyelitis, including infection of the small bones of the hands and feet; liver and lung abscesses; and granulomatous lesions of major organs which fail to resolve, for example sinusitis, antral obstruction of the stomach causing vomiting, and obstructive uropathy.

CGD is a defect in the neutrophil whereby it is unable to kill ingested bacteria. This defect is due to a failure of the neutrophil to activate one or more oxidases to consume oxygen to produce superoxide or hydrogen peroxide following phagocystosis. Hydrogen peroxide stimulates the hexose monophosphate shunt and halides are produced. The interaction of reactive oxygen molecules, myeloperoxidase and halides within phagocytic vacuoles results in effective killing of catalase-containing bacteria. These are staphylococci and enteric bacteria, particularly *Serratia marcescens*. Fungal infections, especially candida and aspergillus, are also common.

CGD is best diagnosed by: (1) the NBT test, when polymorphs demonstrate an inability to reduce NBT; (2) the absence of a respiratory burst, as shown by absent chemiluminescence or iodination, and (3) marked reduction in bacterial killing capacity.

When considering a child with multiple infections, all forms of immunodeficiency disorders should be considered, i.e. total or subclass immunoglobulin deficiency; complement deficiency; T and/or B lymphocyte deficiency or functional defect; neutrophil number, morphology or function deficit. In this case, immunoglobulin, complement and lymphocyte levels are apparently normal; normal antibody levels and PHA response indicate normal T and B function.

Neutrophil function is divided into numbers and morphology

(no remarks are made of film abnormality); mobilization–intramuscular ACTH should increase the peripheral blood neutrophil count by 25% after 6 hours; chemotaxis tests–Boyden's chamber or skin window techniques; adhesion tests either using monoclonal antibodies to identify surface adherence proteins or functional by passing blood through a nylon wool column; phagocytosis–tested by assaying the rate of uptake of opsonized latex particles by the neutrophils. Finally oxidative metabolism results in bacterial killing. Tests´ include the NBT test, chemiluminescence and specific bacterial killing tests for staphylococci, *Escherichia coli* or candida. Certain enzymes such as myeloperoxidase, glucose-6-phosphate dehydrogenase (G6PD), glutathione peroxidase and tuftsin aid bacterial killing, therefore can cause a variable disease pattern if deficient, candidiasis is common.

CGD is sex linked in 75% of patients, autosomal recessive in 20%. Differential diagnosis is with other neutrophil defects, in particular morphological neutrophil abnormalities, e.g. Chédiak–Higashi syndrome and lactoferrin deficiency; mobility disorders, e.g. lazy leukocyte syndome, Schwachman's syndrome where there is also exocrine pancreatic insufficiency and poor growth, and hyper-IgE syndrome in which both catalase-negative and positive organisms predominate. Opsonization or adhesion defects cause sepsis from a wide variety of bacteria such as pneumococcus, streptococcus, meningococcus and *Haemophilus influenzae*. These are all unusual causes for infection in CGD since they are catalase-negative organisms and produce their own hydrogen peroxide, thus assisting their demise within the neutrophil. Bacterial killing defects and enzyme deficiencies have already been discussed.

It must always be remembered that impaired immunity may be secondary to intercurrent or chronic illness, e.g. rheumatoid arthritis, SLE, drugs, tuberculosis, toxoplasmosis or malnutrition.

The neurological lesion described is consistent with anterior wedging of the spinal cord at about T3–4. This is because the arms have intact power and sensation and are supplied from C5–T1. T2 supplies the axilla and is the first intercostal nerve. Since this patient is unable to sit without support, this suggests gross interference with trunk musculature supplied from T2–L3. Joint position sense and coarse touch are carried in the posterior columns of the spinal cord and are intact, while temperature and pain fibres travel in the spinothalamic pathways in the anterior and lateral columns and are not mentioned as being present. Further investigation of the extent of the lesion should be obtained with spinal X-rays which showed collapse of the vertebral bodies of T2–4, and a myelogram or MRI scan to demonstrate the level of block. With such marked paraplegia immediate action is necessary to try to decompress the lesion. This can be done surgically, but active treatment of the aspergillus is most important. Amphotericin is still the only really active agent against aspergillus despite claims made on behalf of other antifungal agents. Since the polymorphs in CGD have defective fungal killing, infusions of white cells may help to clear infection in conjunction with appropriate antimicrobial therapy.

Further reading

Brett, E. M. (1991). *Paediatric Neurology*. Spinal Cord Tumours, pp. 511–24. (Edinburgh; Churchill Livingstone)

Haeney, M. (1991). The detection and management of primary immunodeficiency. In *Recent Advances in Paediatrics* no. 9. Ed. by T. J. David, pp. 21–37. (Edinburgh; Churchill Livingstone)

Landing, B. H. and Shirkey, H. S. (1957). A syndrome of recurrent infection and infiltration of the viscera by pigmented lipid histiocytes. *Pediatrics*, **20**, 431.

Watson, J. G. and Bird, A. G. (1990). *Handbook of Immunological Investigations in Children*, pp. 7–44, 214–40. (London; Butterworths)

Case 22

Answers

1. (a) McCune–Albright's syndrome.
   (b) Neurofibromatosis.
   (c) Child sex abuse.
2. (a) Skeletal survey.
   (b) Gonadotrophins.
   (c) LHRH stimulation test.

Discussion

The child presents with isolated vaginal bleeding for which local causes have been excluded by physical examination and EUA. This does not exclude child sex abuse, neither does a negative reflex anal dilatation but is indicative that repeated physical abuse is an unlikely diagnosis. She is of tall stature and has an advanced bone age, so premature menarche and precocious puberty should be considered. Some 85–90% of females displaying precocious puberty have no underlying pathology and are assumed to be constitutional. However, it is most unusual for vaginal bleeding to be the presenting symptom, whereas sexual precocity secondary to McCune–Albright's syndrome characteristically presents with vaginal bleeding. Café au lait spots and polyostotic fibrous dysplasia are two other commonly associated features of this syndrome. Neurofibromatosis is another possible diagnosis.

Confirmation of McCune–Albright's syndrome would be gained by detecting the fibrotic lesions on X-ray. Both diseases are assumed to act centrally to cause sexual precocity. Gonadatrophins will be consistently high and stimulation with LHRH should evoke an adult response.

Fibrous dysplasia of bone is subdivided into three types: monostotic, involving one bone only; polyostotic, and polyostotic accompanied by café au lait spots and sexual precocity (McCune–Albright's syndrome).

Monostotic may affect any bone, but frequently involves femur, tibia, rib or facial bone. The polyostotic variety may be segmental, involving several bones in one limb. In McCune–Albright's syndrome the café au lait spots, which have an irregular outline, may be distributed over the affected limb.

McCune–Albright's syndrome affects more females than males and is caused by spontaneous mutation; no female has produced an affected offspring. Sexual precocity is the normal endocrine feature, but cases of hyperthyroidism and diabetes mellitus have been described. The disease often presents in infancy with fractures, but may become apparent as late as the fourth decade. Multiple fractures may result in deformity correctable only by surgery. Curettage and bone grafting of the lesions may be beneficial, especially in the adult as the lesions tend to stabilize in adult life. Rarely, sarcomatous change supervenes.

Precocious puberty, defined as the appearance of secondary sexual characteristics before 8 years in a female and 10 years in a male, or the menarche before 10 years, can be classified as central when the hypothalamus or pituitary gland is assumed to be affected, or peripheral when caused by hormone-secreting tumours. Miscellaneous causes include hypothyroidism and exogenous hormones. The majority of males but only 10–15% of females have underlying pathology.

Central causes include cerebral tumours, such as pineal tumours in males, tumours of the hypothalamus and of the floor of the third ventricle and neurofibromatosis, also meningitis, encephalitis, cysts and hydrocephalus. Breast development and pubic hair usually appear before menstruation and in males, both the penis and testes are enlarged. Stature is initially tall and bone age considerably advanced, resulting in eventual small stature. Gonadotrophin levels will be high and the LHRH stimulation test will give an adult response.

Underlying pathology should be sought, especially in males and very young females. If the cause is constitutional, puberty can be suppressed with medroxyprogesterone or cyproterone acetate.

Peripheral causes include ovarian, testicular and adrenal tumours and gonadotrophin-secreting tumours. Masses may be palpated abdominally or rectally, but it must be remembered that ovarian cysts can be induced by central causes. Tall stature and advanced bone age tend to be less marked than in central causes; the penis enlarges, but the testes remain infantile. Except in gonadotrophin-secreting tumours, gonadotrophin levels will be less and sex hormone metabolite levels high; in all tumours an LHRH stimulation test will return a prepubertal result. Management is to delineate and remove the tumours.

Further reading

Carani, C., Pacchioni, C., Baldini, A. and Zini, D. (1988). Effects of cyproterone acetate, LHRH agonist and ovarian surgery in McCune–Albright syndrome with precocious puberty and galactorrhea. *Journal of Endocrinological Investigation*, 11, 419–23.

Usala, A. L. and Blumer, J. L. (1989). Pharmacology of new hormonal therapies in the treatment of pediatric endocrine disorders. *Pediatric Clinics of North America*, 36, 1157–82.

Wheeler, M. D. and Styne, D. M. (1990). Diagnosis and managment of precocious puberty. *Pediatric Clinics of North America*, 37, 1255–71.

Case 23

Answers

1. Haemolytic uraemic syndrome.

2. (a) Convulsions.
   (b) Hypertension.
   (c) Cardiac failure.
   (d) Acute cortical necrosis, renal failure.
   (e) Neurological impairment, i.e. coma/decerebrate rigidity/ hemiparesis.
   (f) Retinal haemorrhages.
3. Fibrin deposition and thrombi in small blood vessels (microangiopathic haemolytic anaemia).

Discussion

From the initial history and examination this child could have haemolytic uraemic syndrome (HUS), intussusception, septicaemia, Henoch–Schönlein purpura, haemolytic crisis, typhoid or poisoning. However, when the investigations are reviewed, thrombocytopenia does not usually occur in these conditions unless disseminated intravascular coagulopathy (DIC) has occurred, whereas it is the normal finding in HUS. DIC is ruled out by the normal fibrinogen assay and thrombin time. In HUS, observations suggest that intravascular coagulation occurs in every patient, but is an initial, very transient phenomenon. Since most children are seen a few days after onset, the most frequent findings are high levels of fibrinogen and some coagulation factors, occurring as a rebound phenomena. About 50% of children do have a prolonged prothrombin time related to a decrease of factor II (prothrombin). Further episodes of DIC may occur but this is unusual; the damage is generally done at the onset. Thrombocytopenia persists for 7–15 days and is followed by a progressive increase in the platelet count.

Pathologically fibrin thrombi develop in small blood vessels, particularly capillaries, with the kidney as a particular target. Linear deposits of fibrin are found on the endothelial surface of the glomerular capillaries, thrombosing them and causing acute renal failure of varying degrees, depending on the percentage of glomeruli affected. In this case renal impairment is reflected in not only the raised urea, which could be accounted for by dehydration, but also the raised creatinine. Going back to the differential diagnoses, detailed above, renal impairment is unlikely unless there has been an episode of hypotension, or direct renal damage from toxin, haemoglobulinuria or proliferative glomerulonephritis.

The same thrombotic process occurring in the CNS produces mild manifestations in approximately half the patients, with irritability, tremor, ataxia and drowsiness. In these cases meningitis and encephalitis would be further differential diagnoses. However, in some patients the problems are more severe, with convulsions, coma, focal neurological signs, decerebrate rigidity, transient hemiparesis, nystagmus and respiratory depression. Retinal haemorrhages are seen in a third of patients. Subdural haematomas are unusual.

Anaemia is usually severe from the onset with extreme pallor. This, with the renal impairment and damage, causes the hypervolaemic cardiac failure and hypertension seen in these patients. Anaemia obviously occurs after haemolytic crisis and occasionally in septicaemia, poisoning or typhoid, but would not be expected in Henoch–Schönlein purpura or intussusception.

Haematuria and proteinuria always occur in this illness but when found may indicate other renal pathology–such as post-streptococcal nephritis, Henoch–Schönlein nephritis and other nephritides, e.g. that associated with SLE. Massive haematuria is present in only 10% of patients with HUS; hyaline, granular and epithelial casts are also found in the urine. These findings should help differentiate HUS from non-renal pathologies.

Further reading

Arbus, G. S. and Farine, M. (1986). Acute renal failure in children. In *Clinical Paediatric Nephrology*, Ed. by R. J. Postlethwaite, pp. 197–208. (Bristol; Wright)
Fong, J. S. C. *et al.* (1982). Haemolytic uraemic syndrome: current concepts and management. *Paediatrics Clinics of North America*, **29**, 835–56.
Levin, M. and Barratt, T. M. (1984). Haemolytic uraemic syndrome. *Archives of Disease in Childhood*, **59**, 397–400.

Case 24

Answers

1. TBM.
2. (a) Lumbar puncture. CSF: cells and cytocentrifuge, culture, Ziehl–Neelsen stain, protein and sugar levels.
   (b) Mantoux test.

    (c) Gastric washings.
    (d) CT scan.
    (e) Skull X-rays.
    (f) EEG.
3. (a) Hydrocephalus.
    (b) Convulsions.
    (c) Hypothalamic disturbances, e.g. inappropriate ADH secretion.
    (d) Cranial nerve palsies.
    (e) Spinal cord block.
4. (a) Space-occupying lesion.
    (b) Drug intoxication.
    (c) Viral meningitis.
    (d) Encephalitis.
    (e) Meningeal spread of a systemic disease, e.g. disseminated malignancy, SLE, sarcoid.

Discussion

This child's history could fit with any one of the differential diagnoses in answer 4. The features that make TBM the most likely are the gradual onset with increasing irritability and drowsiness, change of character, lethargy and mild pyrexia–i.e. stage 1 TBM in which the symptoms are fairly non-specific–but these together with hilar enlargement on the chest X-ray make it the most likely diagnosis. The absence of focal signs and raised intracranial pressure make a space-occupying lesion less likely, especially with this length of history. Focal signs such as cranial nerve palsies (particularly oculomotor) and hemiparesis occur in viral encephalitis and space-occupying lesion. These are also the features of stage 2 TBM, as are persistent headaches, drowsiness, neck stiffness, increasing confusion, tremulousness and involuntary movements.

These complications can make TBM very difficult to differentiate from space-occupying lesions, such as subdural haematoma and cerebral abscess also viral encephalitis. An EEG in encephalitis may show characteristic features and sometimes a focal abnormality. A CT scan would be more helpful in differentiating a space-occupying lesion. A focal lesion may be seen in herpes encephalitis, but in other encephalitides a CT scan is unrewarding. In TBM some degree of ventricular enlargement may be present. Sometimes patients present with convulsions at the onset; this particularly happens before the age of 2 years.

CSF count in viral encephalitis, viral meningitis and cerebral abscess may mimic TBM in the early stages, i.e. polymorpho-nuclear leukocytes, but later changing almost entirely to a lymphocytosis. Usually the cell count rises to 400×10^6/litre and the protein concentration to 0.8–4.0 g/litre, while the glucose level falls, sometimes to zero. Ziehl–Neelsen stain is required to identify tubercle bacilli in the CSF and often they are found only after a prolonged diligent search. There are no pathognomonic changes in the CSF in viral encephalitis.

To diagnose tuberculosis, a Mantoux test should be carried out and will be positive in approximately 80% of cases. Gastric washings in young children may be positive but tubercle bacilli are notoriously difficult to obtain from young children. Chest X-ray is abnormal in about 75% of cases; skull X-rays are unlikely to show any abnormality.

Complications in TBM occur as a result of infection of the meninges, e.g. arachnoiditis, and arteritis causing ischaemia and infarction of areas of the brain or spinal cord. As a result of exudate the CSF circulation may be blocked at the aqueduct of Sylvius or the outlet foramina from the fourth ventricle, causing non-communicating hydrocephalus, or around the basal arteries, causing communicating hydrocephalus. The hypothalamus may be damaged, and inappropriate ADH secretion is a well-recog-nized complication. The arachnoiditis may mechanically strangu-late any of the cranial nerves passing through it, and at a lower level in the spinal cord, cauda equina and spinal root damage may result in a variety of radiculospinal manifestations. Arteritis may also produce a great number of clinical manifestations depending on which part of the CNS is rendered ischaemic.

There are other rare but possible diagnoses. First, any child who presents with an unusual history for which no cause can be found should be screened for drug ingestion. The child may have eaten some poisons or drugs, but the parents may also be guilty of deliberately poisoning the child (Münchausen's syndrome by proxy). Secondly, there may have been meningeal spread of a systemic disease–malignancy or CNS leukaemia being the most likely in a child of this age. Cytocentrifugation of the CSF to look at the cells should aid diagnosis.

Further reading

Brett, E. M. (1991). *Paediatric Neurology*, pp. 619–31, 701–12. (Edinburgh; Church-ill Livingstone)

Meadow, R. (1984). Factitious illness: the hinterland of child abuse. In *Recent Advances in Paediatrics* Ed. by R. Meadow. no. 7, pp. 217–31. (Edinburgh; Churchill Livingstone)

Parsons, M. (1988). *Tuberculous Meningitis*. (Oxford; Oxford University Press)

Case 25

Answers

1. 1 week.
2. Skeletal survey.

Discussion

Transverse fractures in the long bones are usually caused by a direct blow to the limbs; spiral fractures are the normal result of accidental injury. However, there are reports of transverse fractures of the humeri caused by sudden jerking of the upper limbs during play. It is likely, however, that the accident described by the mother would produce a spiral fracture; non-accidental injury must, therefore, be considered and a skeletal survey performed. Survey of this child revealed two rib fractures with callus formation, indicating a previous injury. On further questioning mother admitted to the child abuse, which had occurred since the marital disharmony. Non-accidental injury must be strongly suspected in a case of multiple fractures–certainly if the injuries are of different ages–if the explanation is not consistent with the fracture or in certain types of fracture, notably metaphyseal. A small flake of bone is detached at the insertion of muscle or ligament, the injury being caused by shaking or violent longitudinal forces.

Bone pathology, such as osteogenesis imperfecta or Caffey's disease, should be excluded and many would advocate a coagulation screen even in the absence of bruising. Any external injury should be photographed.

The true incidence of child abuse, either physical or emotional, is unknown. It does occur in all social spheres, but only the minority come to medical attention. Several psychological and social surveys have listed factors that predispose to child abuse. A recent survey listed 62 key characteristics which included aspects of the parents' childhood, their attitudes towards each other, their individual childrearing practices and many social factors. It concluded that any family with 15 or more key characteristics was at high risk of child abuse. This family displays several adverse aspects: both parents were young, the accommodation was poor, income was erratic and inadequate and there was recent marital disharmony. The effect of early maternal bonding and breastfeeding is constantly stressed; premature infants separated from their mothers at birth suffer a higher incidence of child abuse, whereas infants breastfed for more than 6 weeks are rarely abused.

Each child abuse case is managed individually; courses of action are to follow up the child at home with frequent visits, or to place the child on the 'child protection' register which ensures regular health visitor or social worker contact. In more serious cases a place of safety order may be obtained and ultimately the child may be placed in care.

Further reading

Cameron, J. M. and Rae, L. J. (eds) (1975). The radiological diagnosis. In *Atlas of the Battered Child Syndrome*, p. 25. (London; Churchill Livingstone)

King, J., Diefendorf, D., Apthorp, J., Negrete, V. F. and Carlson, M. (1988). Analysis of 429 fractures in 189 battered children. *Journal of Pediatric Orthopedics*, **8**, 585–9.

Silverman, F.N. (1990). The limbs. In *Essentials of Caffey's Pediatric X-Ray Diagnosis*, Ed. by F. N. Silverman and J. P. Kuhn. pp. 911–30. (Chicago; Year Book Medical Publishers)

Case 26

Answers

1. Langerhans cell histiocytosis (Hand–Schüller–Christian disease).
2. (a) Skeletal survey.
   (b) Bone marrow microscopy and staining.
   (c) Electron microscopy.

Discussion

This child presents with two of the three classic features of Hand–Schüller–Christian disease–diabetes insipidus and proptosis–the third, lytic bone lesions, can be demonstrated clinically in the skull and on skeletal survey. He also had a typical skin rash which, although more a feature of Letterer–Siwe disease, may be the presenting feature in Hand–Schüller–Christian disease. Hypothyroidism and renal pathology are unlikely on the investigative results. Growth hormone deficiency may present at this age but does not explain the clinical signs and symptoms.

Histiocytosis X has now been reclassified as three histiocytosis syndromes: Langerhans cell histiocytosis; histiocytoses of mononuclear phagocytes other than Langerhans cells; malignant histiocytic disorders. The previous classification of Hand–Schüller–Christian, Letterer–Siwe and eosinophilic granuloma are now all within the group of Langerhans cell histiocytosis. The previous classification depended largely on physical position. The classification is now on cell type, specific microscopic appearance, enzyme stains and electron microscopic abnormalities being required for a definitive diagnosis. Langerhans cell histiocytosis is not considered to represent a malignant change and prognosis is generally good. Indeed over-intensive therapy may be detrimental. However, those children who have evidence of organ failure have a poorer prognosis.

Diabetes insipidus may remit with therapy; if not, vasopressin (DDAVP) must be administered to the patient.

Further reading

Broadbent, V., Gadner, H., Komp, D.M. and Ladisch, S. (1989). Histiocytosis syndromes in children: II. Approach to the clinical and laboratory evaluation of children with Langerhans cell histiocytosis. *Medical and Pediatric Oncology*, **17**, 492–5.

McLelland, J., Broadbent, V., Yeomans, E., Malone, M. and Pritchard, J. (1990). Langerhans cell histiocytosis: the case for conservative treatment. *Archives of Disease in Childhood*, **65**, 301–3.

Raney, R. B. and D'Angio, G. J. (1989). Langerhans' cell histiocytosis (histiocytosis X): experience at the Children's Hospital of Philadelphia, 1970–1984. *Medical and Pediatric Oncology*, **17**, 20–8.

Writing Group of the Histiocyte Society. (1987). Histiocytosis syndromes in childhood. *Lancet*, **1**, 208–9.

Case 27

Answers

1. (a) Intraventricular haemorrhage (IVH).
   (b) Pneumothorax.
2. (a) Transillumination of the hemithoraces with a cold light source.
   (b) Diagnostic tap of the suspected hemithorax.
   (c) Chest X-ray.
   (d) Cerebral ultrasound.

Discussion

The immediate possibility which should be excluded in this infant is the position and patency of the endotracheal tube; these variables were excluded, but the child did not respond. Inhalation is unlikely as the gastric aspirate was negligible; infection is also unlikely as this generally leads to gradual deterioration and the child was on antibiotics. Pulmonary haemorrhage is a possibility, but no blood was seen during intubation and air entry was noted to be good. The two most likely diagnoses are, therefore, IVH and pneumothorax.

If a pneumothorax is suspected, transillumination of the hemithoraces allows immediate diagnosis and treatment. Chest X-ray may well take too long so a diagnostic tap of the suspected side, using such clues as deviation of the trachea, displacement of the apex beat and differential air entry, may be given. The last sign, however, may not be as useful, as chests sounds are well-transmitted in the neonate.

IVH is common in this age group and the incidence is increased by IPPV. There are four categories of IVH: (1) a small subependymal haemorrhage, usually with slight or no clinical symptoms; (2) with extension into the ipsilateral ventricle there may be little clinical disturbance; (3) with blood in the contralateral ventricle; and (4) with dilatation of the ventricles. The last two categories usually have marked clinical symptoms and may well be fatal.

The aetiology of the IVH is controversial. There is still debate as to whether the haemorrhage emanates from the capillaries or from the venous side, but there is agreement that the neonatal lack of autoregulation of cerebral blood flow is a major factor.

Invasive diagnostic techniques are no longer justified as immediate diagnosis does not influence treatment and non-invasive techniques such as CT scanning and ultrasound are now reliable. Diagnosis is important for the long-term management of these children, as awareness allows informed decisions as to treatment of complications such as hydrocephalus.

Recent work has suggested that the use of vitamin E given early in susceptible infants may reduce the incidence of IVH.

Further reading

Chiswick, M., Gladman, G., Sinha, S., Toner, N. and Davies, J. (1991). Vitamin E supplementation and periventricular hemorrhage in the newborn. *American Journal of Clinical Nutrition*, **53**, (suppl 1), 370S–2S.

de Vries, L.S., Larroche, J-C. and Levene, M.I . (1988). Germinal matrix haemorrhage and intraventricular haemorrhage. In *Fetal and Neonatal Neurology and Neurosurgery*, Ed. by M. I. Levene, M. J. Bennett and J. Punt, pp. 312–25. (London; Churchill Livingstone)

Trounce, J. Q., Levene, M. I. (1988). Ultrasound imaging of the neonatal brain. In *Fetal and Neonatal Neurology and Neurosurgery*, Ed. by M. I. Levene, M. J. Bennett and J. Punt, pp. 139–48. (London; Churchill Livingstone)

Case 28

Answers

1. β-Thalassaemia major.
2. Chorionic villus sampling for fetal DNA analysis.
3. (a) Transfusion problem–sensitization to HLA and minor blood group antigens.
   (b) Iron overload.
   (c) Hypersplenism.
   (d) Folate deficiency.

Discussion

The diagnosis is β-thalassaemia major. This condition occurs in children of parents who are heterozygotes for the β-thalassaemia gene. In this disorder adult Hb, which consists of two α chains and two β chains, cannot be synthesized. The disorder is one of the regulation of β chain synthesis rather than an absence of the β chain genes, and several types of genetic defects are known to occur which determine how much α chain is synthesized. In $\beta°$-thalassaemia, which is the most severe, there is no Hb A production, while in $\beta+$ and β intermedia there is some Hb A production. The consequences of the failure to synthesize Hb A are: a profound hypochromic microcytic anaemia due to failure of red cell haemoglobinization, increased destruction of defective red cells giving rise to splenomegaly and mild jaundice, and a compensatory increase in erythropoiesis resulting in extension of the red marrow throughout the bony medulla, with bony expansion especially prominent in the facial bones and skull, and circulating erythroblasts. The predominant Hb synthesized in thalassaemia major is Hb F (two γ, two α chains) and Hb A2 (two δ, two α chains). In addition there is an excess of α chains synthesized in the red cell which precipitate within it to produce the appearance of basophilic stippling.

The thalassaemia gene has a high incidence in people of Mediterranean and Far Eastern origin, and thalassaemia major should be suspected in any child of such parents presenting with a profound hypochromic anaemia in the first year of life. The differential diagnosis is hypochromic anaemia due to iron deficiency, or other Hb variants such as Hb Lepore, Hb E+ thalassaemia and α-thalassaemia minor (Hb H disease) which can easily be distinguished by Hb electrophoresis.

The diagnosis is made on the characteristic blood picture of profound hypochromia with microcytes, poikilocytes and ghost-like red cells (leptocytes), together with features of chronic haemolysis: increased unconjugated bilirubin, circulating nucleated red cells, leukocytosis and occasionally reticulocytosis. The diagnosis is confirmed by Hb electrophoresis. There is a predominance of Hb F, Hb A2 is often marginally raised, and there is a variable amount of Hb A production according to the exact gene defect. This patient has $\beta+$ thalassaemia since there is some Hb A production. Further investigations, such as estimating the rates of β and α chain synthesis in the erythroblasts, are usually only applicable as research procedures. Following family studies, antenatal diagnosis may be possible with chorionic villus sampling and DNA analysis.

The management is regular blood transfusion to keep the Hb in the range of over 10 g/100 ml; this will require transfusions every 3–4 weeks. Patients will rapidly develop problems associated with chronic transfusion treatment–sensitization to HLAs requires the careful selection of blood free of minor antigens by the transfusion centre. Desferrioxamine given with transfusion and administered subcutaneously overnight up to 5 days a week continually should be instituted as soon as regular transfusions are commenced. Measurements of serum ferritin will identify whether iron overload is occurring, and folic acid supplements may be necessary in some patients with excessive erythropoiesis. Occasionally splenomegaly may be a problem requiring splenectomy to reduce haemolysis. Splenectomy should be delayed as long as possible to reduce the risk of post-splenectomy immune defects, when pneumococcal and *Haemophilus influenzae* septicaemia can occur. Pneumococcal antigen vaccination before splenectomy is helpful in reducing this risk.

Further reading

Weatherall, D. J. and Clegg, J. B. (1981). *Thalassaemia Syndrome*. (Oxford; Blackwell Scientific Publications)

Ohene-Frempong, K. and Schwartz, E. (1980). Clinical features of thalassaemia. *Pediatric Clinics of North America*, Vol. 27, Part 2, 403–20. (Philadelphia; W. B. Saunders)

Case 29

Answers

1. (a) CT scan.
    (b) MRI scan.
    (c) Blood pressure.
    (d) Skull X-ray.
    (e) Viral titres.
2. Pseudotumor cerebri (benign intracranial hypertension) secondary to otitis media.
3. Reduction of the raised intracranial pressure by:
    (a) Hypertonic solutions.
    (b) Surgical decompression.
    (c) Ventriculoperitoneal shunt.

4. (a) Addison's disease.
   (b) Cushing's disease.
   (c) Hypoparathyroidism.
   (d) Hypothyroidism.
   (e) Tetracyclines.
   (f) Steroids.
   (g) Penicillin.
   (h) Pulmonary encephalopathy.
   (i) Infectious mononucleosis.
   (j) High protein in CSF, e.g. polyneuritis.

Discussion

There are numerous causes of raised intracranial pressure in childhood; however, two aspects of this child's history warrant closer attention. The fall may be relevant, although he was not knocked out and there was no history of head injury. However, the history is too long for either an extradural or acute subdural haemorrhage, both of which should cause signs within 24–36 hours. A skull X-ray should also reveal a fracture.

The other aspect is the otitis media suffered 2 weeks previously. Otitis media may cause a variety of intracranial complications including meningitis and cerebral abscess. However, he had only mild nuchal rigidity and both the tripod and Kernig's signs were negative; he was also apyrexial. CSF analysis and pressure would be useful, but are contraindicated in the presence of signs of raised intracranial pressure. Repeated lumbar punctures have been used to reduce intracranial pressure in benign intracranial hypertension once the diagnosis has been unequivocally established. The period between presentation and the initial infection is also somewhat long. A likely diagnosis is, therefore, otitic hydrocephalus or pseudotumor cerebri. The mechanism for raised intracranial pressure is thought to be non-septic thrombosis of the lateral venous sinus.

The blood pressure can be useful, but if high it may be the cause or the result of the encephalopathy.

Symptoms are those of raised intracranial pressure. There may be a loss of visual acuity from papilloedema and a particularly ominous sign is amaurosis fugax–repeated, transient, episodes of dimming or loss of vision. Diplopia may occur from an abducens palsy. The CSF in this condition is normal except for the grossly raised pressure.

The time span from the original coryza is consistent with a viral encephalitis. The CSF may be normal, but this child is apyrexial, has a normal WBC and no lymphocytosis. A CT scan in encephalitis may reveal cerebral oedema or a localized lesion in herpes encephalitis. In pseudotumor cerebri the scan is either normal or shows small ventricles.

The child has markedly raised intracranial pressure as evidenced by papilloedema and a sixth nerve palsy; urgent treatment is therefore required. Cerebral oedema is not a feature of this syndrome; however, hypertonic solutions may reduce the intracranial pressure rapidly. Other approaches include surgical decompression or a ventriculoperitoneal shunt. However, as the ventricles are normal or small, positioning the shunt may be difficult. This condition may last several months, but usually resolves spontaneously and has a good prognosis. However, there may be loss of visual acuity.

Pseudotumor cerebri may be seen in many diseases, which can be broadly divided into the following categories:

1. Intracranial venous thrombosis.
2. Endocrine disorders.
   (a) Addison's disease.
   (b) Cushing's disease.
   (c) Hypoparathyroidism.
   (d) Hypothyroidism.
3. Vitamins and drugs.
   (a) Vitamin A intoxication.
   (b) Iron deficiency.
   (c) Tetracycline therapy.
   (d) Steroid therapy.
   (e) Penicillin therapy.
4. High CSF protein.
   (a) Polyneuritis.
   (b) Tumours of the cauda equina.
5. Haematological.
   (a) Polycythaemia.
   (b) Infectious mononucleosis.
6. (a) Pulmonary encephalopathy.
   (b) Pickwickian syndrome.
7. Miscellaneous.
   (a) Roseola infantum.
   (b) Sydenham's chorea.
   (c) Familial.
8. Idiopathic.

168

It must be stressed, however, that pseudotumor cerebri is a diagnosis of exclusion in many instances and full investigation of each suspected patient is mandatory.

Further reading

Baker, R. S., Baumann, R. J. and Buncic, J. R. (1989). Idiopathic intracranial hypertension (pseudotumor cerebri) in pediatric patients. *Pediatric Neurology*, **5**, 5–11.

Round, R., Keane, J. R. (1988). The minor symptoms of increased intracranial pressure: 101 patients with benign intracranial hypertension. *Neurology*, **38**, 1461–4.

Case 30

Answers

1. Giardiasis.
2. (a) Warm-stool microscopy × 3.
   (b) Jejunal intubation for biopsy and juice aspiration.
   (c) Barium studies.
   (d) Dietary assessment.
   (e) IgE.
   (f) Liver function tests.

Discussion

This is a child who has followed a normal course for the first 2 years of his life apart from repeated upper respiratory tract infections, which is expected in a child with selective IgA deficiency. With the above history, some diagnoses suggest themselves, such as Crohn's disease, Hirschsprung's disease, coeliac disease, giardiasis, *Campylobacter, Yersinia* or *Cryptosporidium* enterocolitis; and food allergy.

Crohn's disease is a definite possibility with abdominal pain, intermittent diarrhoea, poor growth and weight gain, plus a borderline albumin. Factors against this are its rarity in a 4-year-old child, the lack of blood in the stools and iron-deficiency anaemia; there should also be a raised C-reactive protein or ESR. Diagnosis should be with barium studies and possibly biopsy.

Hirschsprung's disease is unlikely but can be investigated by barium enema, rectal biopsy and anorectal manometry. The infections named above are usually more acute, but chronic problems are sometimes seen. *Campylobacter* and *Cryptosporidium* should be isolated from the stool but serological identification is more reliable for *Yersinia*.

Coeliac disease is unlikely here in view of the normal xylose absorption test results, lack of steatorrhoea and muscle wasting on examination. However, with a history of failure to thrive, a borderline albumin level, diarrhoea and abdominal pain, a jejunal biopsy is always a worthwhile investigation. Food allergy such as cows' milk, protein or egg intolerance may present with a similar history but usually this occurs in infancy and not at the age of 4 years.

Giardia may be found in 16–21% of children's gastrointestinal tracts. The degree of pathogenicity is still in question. There are three types of presentation: first, acute with foul-smelling stools, flatus, abdominal distension but no blood or pus. Secondly, a subacute infection which may last for some months and can mimic hiatus hernia, cholecystitis and hepatitis. It may be associated with failure to thrive and is probably the category that this child fits into. Thirdly, there is chronic infection lasting for years and associated with malabsorption of fat, D-xylose and vitamin B_{12}, similar to tropical sprue. The question always arises as to why some people are symptomatic and others not. Alternative factors may be present, such as hypogammaglobulinaemia, deficiency of secretory IgA, and unusual bacterial flora of the jejunum, or other pathology present in the patient; these may combine synergistically with *Giardia* to cause symptoms. The immunoglobulin abnormalities and possible stasis from constipation might have predisposed this child to giardiasis.

Diagnosis initially should be by microscopy of three warm, concentrated stools. However, the microscopy is positive in only about 30% of patients. Secondly, duodenal intubation with aspiration of jejunal juice may give positive results in about 70% of cases. However, if jejunal biopsy is added, approximately 90% of cases will be diagnosed; this is certainly the most reliable investigation.

In the child, lack of weight gain may be due to poor food intake with an inadequate calorie requirement. Thus a dietary assessment should be done. IgE estimation is not a very good indicator of food allergy, but specific IgE to egg, cows' milk and other foodstuffs may be helpful. Liver function tests are indicated in a child who is unwell, especially with a family history of recent infectious hepatitis. Children often have a subclinical form of this infection.

Further reading

Joss, V. and Brueton, M. (1981). Unsuspected giardiasis. *Lancet*, **ii**, 996.
Manson-Bahr, P. E. C. and Bell, D. R. (1987). *Manson's Tropical Diseases*, pp. 324–7. (London; Baillière Tindall)
Walker-Smith, J. (1988). *Diseases of the Small Intestine in Childhood*, 3rd edn, pp. 315–22. (London; Butterworths)

Case 31

Answers

1. In the endocardium of the right ventricle opposite the ventricular septal defect, where the jet of blood impinges on the ventricular wall.
2. Long-term antibiotics and removal and replacement of the atrioventricular shunt.

Discussion

This child has signs and symptoms of a chronic infection: lethargy, low-grade pyrexia unresponsive to antibiotics and indicative blood film changes. One negative blood culture does not exclude the diagnosis; a series of blood cultures should be taken when the temperature is spiking. Examination revealed a harsh pansystolic murmur at the left sternal edge, indicative of cardiac pathology; subacute bacterial endocarditis is therefore a likely diagnosis. Additional corroborative signs are splenomegaly and retinal haemorrhages.

The endocarditis may be secondary to an infected shunt. If not, the valve will almost certainly have been infected and should be replaced after vigorous antibiotic therapy. Infection of the shunt may be confirmed by direct sampling of CSF from the valve. Also, complement levels and anti-staphylococcal titres may be raised. The distal catheter may be exteriorized, discarding infected CSF and increasing antibiotic efficiency. The infecting organisms are usually bacterial and of low pathogenicity, initiating sporadic bacteraemias and spiking pyrexias. Mycotic emboli produce ubiquitous vascular lesions, most noticeable in the retina–boat-shaped haemorrhage–and under the nails–'splinter haemorrhage'. Renal involvement in bacterial endocarditis is due to deposition of immune complexes. Histology reveals a focal proliferative glomerulonephritis with areas of necrosis. Haematuria and proteinuria may be marked. Shunt nephritis following shunt infection is membranoproliferative glomerulonephritis, also probably caused by immune complexes. Again haematuria and proteinuria are induced and the nephrotic syndrome may occur.

All prostheses are susceptible to infection which, once established, is difficult to eradicate as host defences are unable to act synergistically with antibiotics. Prophylactic antibiotics should be given to cover dental and surgical procedures.

Further reading

de Wardener, H. E. (ed.) (1985). In *The Kidney*, pp. 374, 431. (London; Churchill Livingstone)

Kaplan, E. L. and Shulman, S. T. (1989). Endocarditis. In *Moss' Heart Disease in Infants, Children and Adolescents*, 4th edn. Ed. by F. H. Adams, G. C. Emmanouilides and T. A. Riemenschneider, pp. 719–29. (Baltimore; Williams & Wilkins)

Case 32

Answers

1. Disseminated CNS malignancy.
2. (a) Non-Hodgkin's lymphoma.
   (b) Leukaemia.
   (c) Medulloblastoma.

Discussion

This boy presents with one of the classic signs of raised intracranial pressure, namely sixth nerve palsy. It is unaccompanied by the typical symptoms, headache and vomiting. The sixth nerve palsy could be an isolated lesion but there are other signs and symptoms to account for. These are the upper lip tingling, suggesting involvement of the fifth nerve sensory nucleus which has a long tail descending to the upper medulla; and the eighth nerve deafness with minimal intention tremor on the same side, suggesting a lesion in the cerebellar pontine angle.

The symptoms of later onset are impossible to put down to a posterior fossa lesion. Upper motor neuron signs in the legs with nothing similar in the arms makes a pyramidal or cord lesion likely, involving the motor tracts, i.e. anterior, while urinary retention and chest pain may be secondary to root lesions. The combination of two out of three of the following problems–truncal pain, urinary symptoms and walking difficulties, often with a change in character of the child–virtually always heralds serious CNS disease in my experience. The signs are best explained by disseminated disease, most likely malignancy in the CNS. In children non-Hodgkin's lymphoma, leukaemia and brain tumours may produce such a clinical picture. Early papilloedema may often be present but is not a necessity in such a disseminated picture.

Some primary CNS tumours disseminate via the CSF, namely medulloblastoma and occasionally ependymoma, but these usually present with signs resulting from the primary lesion in the posterior fossa, i.e. ataxia plus raised intracranial pressure. Medulloblastoma is more common in younger age groups, particularly 1–5 years. Other 'common' brain tumours are astrocytomes and gliomas. Malignancies such as neuroblastoma or rhabdomyosarcoma may spread directly or indirectly to the CNS and surrounding bony structures, causing very varied symptoms and signs.

Non-Hodgkin's lymphoma arises in lymphatic tissue in 80% of cases, either nodal or extranodal. There is early haematogenous and lymphatic spread, so that the primary site may not always be apparent. The commonest sites for tumour growth are in the head and neck, as an anterior mediastinal mass and in the abdomen with or without intestinal obstruction. Bone pain, marrow infiltration and general symptoms such as fever, weight loss and fatigue may occur. CNS involvement occurs in a significant number of patients–up to one-third in some series–with raised intracranial pressure and cranial nerve involvement. Interestingly, leukaemia may result in a similar clinical picture with CNS involvement, and approximately 33% of patients with non-Hodgkin's lymphoma develop leukaemia.

There are other causes of disseminated CNS disease which should be considered such as tuberose sclerosis, neurofibromatosis, sarcodosis, SLE and polyarteritis nodosa, but the associated stigmata should be present to assist diagnosis.

The CT scans were negative, probably because of the diffuse pattern of the malignancy with small deposits low in the posterior fossa and upper cervical cord, a region difficult to define. A myelogram or preferably an MRI scan would now be the investigation of choice.

Further reading

Brett, E. M. (1991). *Paediatric Neurology*, pp. 511–24, 701–12. (Edinburgh; Churchill Livingstone)

Cohen, M. E. and Duffner, P. K. (1985). Current therapy in childhood brain tumours. *Neurological Clinics: Paediatric Neurology*. Vol. 3, Part 1, pp. 147–64. (Philadelphia; W. B. Saunders)

Mott, M. G. (1979). The presentation, management and prognosis of solid tumours in childhood. In *Topics in Paediatrics*. I. *Haematology and Oncology*, Ed. by P. H. Morris Jones, pp. 51–65. (London; Pitman)

Case 33

Answers

1. (a) Vitamin D-resistant or dependent rickets.
   (b) Urinary tract infection.
2. Autosomal recessive.
3. 1-alphahydroxycholecalciferol.

Discussion

When confronted with a case of rickets, the various causes must be systematically considered and excluded one by one. This child does not appear to have been malnourished from the history and, as a regular attender at clinic, probably would have been given vitamin supplementation. Malabsorption certainly is a possibility with mild iron deficiency and a borderline xylose tolerance, but the normal albumin and stool microscopy makes this unlikely. Liver function tests are normal, which indicates normal hepatocellular function. Thus hepatic hydroxylation of vitamin D should be intact. If sophisticated laboratory facilities are available, 25-hydroxycholecalciferol can be measured.

The next step in the pathway is the kidney. There are several problems that may occur. First, there are the renal tubular defects, both proximal and distal. In proximal defects there is reduced tubular reabsorption of bicarbonate, resulting in a low plasma bicarbonate with a surprisingly high urinary pH. The Fanconi syndrome consists of proximal renal tubular acidosis (RTA), glycosuria, aminoaciduria, hypokalaemia and hypophosphataemia secondary to decreased phosphate reabsorption, giving rise to bone disease. This is not the picture here. Distal tubular acidosis results from an inability to excrete appropriate amounts of acid with an insufficient H^+ gradient. This child is able to cope with an acid-loading test, i.e. the urine pH is less than 5.8. Hyperphosphaturia also occurs in hypophosphataemic rickets, in which aminoaciduria does not occur; the condition has an X-linked dominant inheritance. This is unlikely because plasma phosphate is just within the normal range and urinary phosphate output is normal.

Renal hydroxylation of 25-hydroxycholecalciferol may be defective, either secondary to renal failure (not in this case, as the urea result is normal). There are two types of vitamin D-resistant rickets, type I, where the hydroxylation enzyme appears to be missing, and type II, where there is end-organ resistance to 1,25-hydroxycholecalciferol. If measured, the 25-hydroxycholecalciferol is usually normal, with a raised parathormone due to secondary hyperparathyroidism. Patients generally have low to normal plasma phosphate values and a low calcium level and may present with tetany, aminoaciduria and high alkaline phosphatase activity. This boy does not have all the features, but this is the most likely diagnosis. His parents were first cousins and this fits with the autosomal recessive inheritance of this condition.

Treatment used to be with large doses of vitamin D, but now that 1-α-hydroxycholecalciferol, the synthetic analogue of 1,25-dihydroxy vitamin D, is available, this is usually used, especially as it is short-acting, thus causing less hypercalcaemia.

This child also has a urinary tract infection as an incidental finding, but this had no relationship to the original disease.

Further reading

Fraser, D. and Scriver, C. R. (1976). Familial forms of vitamin D resistant rickets revisited. *American Journal of Clinical Nutrition*, **29**, 1315.

Mughal, Z. and Postlethwaite, R. J. (1986). *Clinical Paediatric Nephrology*, Ed. by Postlethwaite, R. J., pp. 109–21. (Bristol; Wright)

Case 34

Answers

1. (a) Riley–Day syndrome (familial dysautonomia).
   (b) Krabbe's leukodystrophy.
   (c) Perlizaeus–Merzbacher leukodystrophy.
2. (a) Intradermal histamine response.
   (b) Methacholine eye drops.
   (c) Urinary VMA and homomandelic acid (HMA).
   (d) Serum dopamine-β-hydroxylase.
   (e) White cell enzymes.

Discussion

This child presents with diffuse psychological and physical signs. She exhibits some features of failure to thrive: poor weight gain, irritability with difficult feeding and vomiting. She also displays psychological and neurological signs: temper tantrums with breath-holding episodes (which are normally manifest at 9–12 months) and absent tendon and corneal reflexes, with diminished tear production and corneal ulceration. These signs developed after 4 months of normal life, suggesting either a metabolic or a degenerative disorder. Gut dysfunction alone would not explain the diverse neurological problems.

The combination of impaired sensation (absent coneal reflex) diminished tear production, temper tantrums, smooth tongue (loss of fungiform papillae) and absent tendon reflexes is highly suggestive of Riley–Day syndrome (familial dysautonomia); however, both Krabbe's and Perlizaeus–Merzbacher leukodystrophies may present at this age with highly variable signs. Perlizaeus–Merzbacher disease is less likely as hyper-reflexia rather than hyporeflexia obtains.

Postencephalitis syndromes or cerebral sclerosis tend to affect the pyramidal and extrapyramidal systems more than the autonomic and sensory pathways.

Riley–Day syndrome (familial dysautonomia) is a rare, recessively inherited disease, almost exclusively affecting those of Eastern European Jewish descent. The infant often has intrauterine growth retardation, but thereafter develops normally until several months old, when signs develop. Muscle inco-ordination results in difficulty in deglutition, gagging and aspiration which, with excess bronchial secretions, produces repeated chest infections, often of sufficient severity to induce cor pulmonale. Excess salivation, causing drooling and hyperhidrosis, occurs, but tear production is either markedly compromised or absent.

Other autonomic abnormalities include labile hypertension, or orthostatic hypertension, periodic fever and blotching of the skin, especially when excited.

Peripheral sensory dysfunction causes reduction or absence of pain sensation with skin lesions and asymptomatic fractures, absent corneal sensation, taste and deep tendon reflexes.

Histological examination of the peripheral nerve fibres demonstrates reduction both of unmyelinated fibres carrying pain, temperature and taste and of large myelinated fibres carrying afferent impulses from muscle spindles.

Diagnosis is clinical and biochemical. Intradermal histamine produces a much diminished response. Methacholine, which detects denervation hypersensitivity of the iris, constricts the pupil within 10 min if positive; 25% of the older children lack dopamine β-hydroxylase, which catalyses dopamine to noradrenaline. There is, therefore, a reduction in urinary VMA from noradrenaline metabolism with associated increase in HMA from dopamine.

Treatment is supportive only: treatment of the recurrent chest infections, artificial tears and prevention of injuries. Chlorpromazine has been used with moderate success to control the hypertensive and vomiting episodes. The prognosis is hopeless–death usually occurs in childhood.

The hallmark of Krabbe's or globoid cell leukodystrophy is a rapidly progressive degeneration of the white matter with an accumulation of galactocerebroside, the result of a probable absence of galactocerebroside-β-galactosidase, resulting in scattered globoid bodies and myelin balls. Symptoms occur at 4–6 months with implacable crying; this is followed by apathy and stupor. Later the musculature stiffens and eventually becomes totally rigid, gavage is therefore necessary for feeding. Deafness, blindness and tonic or clonic fits rapidly supervene. Prognosis is hopeless, death usually occurring within the first year. Just prior to death, the musculature becomes flaccid with paralysis.

Perlizaeus–Merzbacher disease is classified as a lipid storage disorder, but as yet neither the lipid nor enzyme defect have been identified. It is characterized by slow, progressive, universal, symmetrical demyelination of the cerebral white matter, with dense gliosis. The process begins around the ventricles and spreads towards the cortex. Inheritance is either autosomal or sex-linked recessive, but of irregular behaviour. Symptoms become manifest at 3–4 months and are highly variable, but rotary head movements with rotary nystagmus may occur early. Spasticity occurs first in the legs and then the arms with increased tendon reflexes. The inexorable progression of the disease causes abnormal movements, weakness and paralysis with subsequent contractures. Although there is no treatment, these patients can experience a normal life span if nursed adequately.

Further reading

Rilley–Day syndrome
Axelrod, F. B., Porges, R. F. and Sein, M. E. (1987). Neonatal recognition of familial dysautonomia. *Journal of Pediatrics*, **110**, 946–8.
Walton, J. (ed.) (1985). Disorders of the autonomic nervous system. In *Brain's Diseases of the Nervous System*, 9th edn, pp. 599. (Oxford; Oxford University Press)
Krabbe's leukodystrophy
Ford, F. R. (ed.) (1966). Intoxications, metabolic and endocrine disorders. Dietary deficiencies and involving the nervous system. In *Diseases of the Nervous System in Infancy, Childhood and Adolescence*, 5th edn, p. 757. (Illinois; C. C. Thomas)
Perlizaeus–Merzbacher leukodystrophy
Stephenson, J. B. P. and King, M. D. (eds) (1989). *Handbook of Neurological Investigations in Children*, pp. 46, 68, 79, 150, 151, 161, 173, 210, 211, 215. (London; Wright)
Walton, J. (ed.) (1985). Intoxications and metabolic disorders. In *Brain's Diseases of the Nervous System*, 9th edn, pp. 455, 459. (Oxford; Oxford University Press)

Case 35

Answers

1. Catheterization.
2. (a) Full blood count and differential.
   (b) Erect and supine abdominal X-rays.
   (c) Ultrasound.
   (d) Urine culture.
   (e) Blood culture.
   (f) Stool culture.
   (g) Barium enema.
   (h) Indium labelling of WBC with abdominal scan.
3. Pelvic appendix abscess.

Discussion

Initially it appears that this child has a complication of chickenpox, but on closer examination this seems less likely. Chickenpox encephalitis classically starts about 7–10 days after the onset of the rash and affects the cerebellum. To account for the acute retention and constipation, a transverse myelitis would have to be postulated, but the marked pyrexia and second abdominal mass do not fit.

The history given is fairly classic, of an acute appendicitis with vomiting, diarrhoea and colicky lower abdominal pain. In a young child, perforation usually occurs early so that the later stage of constipation is not reached. However, this child's condition appears to settle, only to flare up again with a pyrexia, constipation and a dull mass between the bladder and rectum, with secondary acute urinary retention. A pelvic appendix abscess is the most likely diagnosis since it is best felt rectally and the symptoms and signs fit with the duration of the history.

The most important clinical procedure to carry out is relief of the acute urinary retention, most easily done by catheterization. Following this, investigation should be aimed at establishing the diagnosis as far as possible, and ruling out other possibilities. These are: mesenteric adenitis, which is usually associated with an upper respiratory tract infection and runs a shorter course; an acute exacerbation of Crohn's disease, unlikely because of the lack of previous symptoms and perianal signs; Hirschsprung's disease or chronic constipation which may cause urinary retention secondary to hard faeces, but again unlikely with no previous history; urinary tract infection; gastroenteritis, especially *Yersinia enterocolitica*; chronic intussusception, which could fit with the earliest symptoms; lastly, ovarian tumours such as a dermoid which may undergo torsion or become infected and prolapse into the pouch of Douglas.

Investigations such as blood, urine and stool cultures should be done to establish the presence of any pathogens. FBC may help to show infection with a high polymorph count, a left shift and toxic granulation. Plain abdominal X-rays, erect and supine, may show abnormal gas pattern of the bowel in the pelvic area with some localized fluid levels. Ultrasound scan should delineate the mass, but rarely a barium enema will be necessary to view the position of the caecum and non-filling appendix. An indium isotope scan for labelled WBC should show a 'hot spot' over the abscess area, but this investigation has limited availability and specificity; laparotomy is the best answer.

Further reading

Black, I. A. (1979). *Paediatric Emergencies*, p. 382. (London; Butterworths)
Nixon, H. and O'Donnell, B. (1992). *Essentials of Paediatric Surgery*. 4th Edn. (Oxford; Butterworth–Heinemann)

Case 36

Answers

1. The frontal sinus.
2. (a) Cerebral oedema.
   (b) Superficial venous cerebral thrombosis.
   (c) Extension of the subdural empyema.
3. (a) CT.
   (b) EEG.
   (c) Burr holes.
   (d) Viral titres.

Discussion

This girl demonstrates the classic history of a frontal sinusitis with frontal pain persisting for several days after the resolution of the coryza. The infection then tracked through the skull to produce a subdural empyema. A small collection of pus was drained but this would not explain the gross oedema of the right hemisphere, the papilloedema or the clinical signs. There are non-specific signs of raised intracranial pressure such as the third and sixth nerve palsies, and specific signs, hemiplegia and hemianopia, which suggest a lesion in the region of the central sulcus. These specific signs could have been caused by gross cerebral oedema, superficial venous thrombophlebitis or extension of the subdural empyema. An extension of the empyema is suggested by her deterioration on the third postoperative day; this was confirmed by a further CT scan. An EEG may be helpful, showing slow wave activity over the lesion; burr holes should reveal a collection of pus. A lumbar puncture is contraindicated, although meningeal extension is possible after operative intervention. If necessary, CSF should be collected from the cisternae.

Common organisms implicated in subdural empyema are pneumococci, *Streptococcus milleri* and anaerobes. The initial infection may have been local, such as sinusitis or otitis media, or distant, as in suppurative lung disease or with a right-to-left vascular shunt.

Three stages of abscess formation are recognized: first, areas of softening and liquefaction appear; secondly these areas coalesce and pus formation occurs. The final stage is reaction around the abscess, localizing the collection. The clinical signs of a cerebral abscess are extraordinarily varied.

Low-grade infection may produce malaise only, the later signs reflecting a space-occupying lesion. A more virulent infection will produce raised intracranial pressure early with cerebral oedema and focal signs such as hemiplegia and cranial nerve palsies. The CSF is usually sterile, but has raised protein and white cell count, predominantly polymorphonuclear leukocytes.

Treatment is a combination of chemotherapy and surgical drainage where possible. All cases are now potentially curable with prompt diagnosis, but in some series a mortality of 40% still occurs.

Further reading

Marshall, W. C. (1983). Infections of the nervous system. In *Paediatric Neurology*, Ed. by E. M. Brett. pp. 522–4. (Edinburgh; Churchill Livingstone)
Stephenson, J. B. P. and King, M. D. (eds). (1989). Acute encephalopathy. In

Handbook of Neurological Investigations in Children, pp. 198–207. (London; Wright)

Walton, J. (ed). (1985). Suppurative encephalitis: intracranial abscess. In *Brain's Diseases of the Nervous System*, 9th edn. pp. 250–3. (Oxford; Oxford University Press)

Case 37

Answers

1. (a) Sweat test.
   (b) Jejunal biopsy.
   (c) Complement breakdown products after cows' milk challenge.
   (d) Stool chymotrypsin activity.
   (e) Stool culture.
   (f) Stool and urine reducing substances.
   (g) Lactose tolerance.
   (h) D-xylose absorption test.
2. (a) Cystic fibrosis.
   (b) Coeliac disease.
   (c) Cows' milk protein intolerance.
   (d) Lactose intolerance.
   (e) Gastroenteritis.

Discussion

The most likely diagnosis in this child is cystic fibrosis. He has had abnormal stools since birth, he is failing to thrive and has a raised respiratory rate with persistent substernal recession. These last two signs, with overexpansion, are often the earliest signs of chest involvement occurring before any radiological changes. A paroxysmal cough culminating in vomiting is characteristic of cystic fibrosis. A similar situation obtains in pertussis, but this child has had two triple immunizations, which reduces the likelihood of pertussis considerably.

Cystic fibrosis is the commonest inherited disease in the UK, occurring in approximately 1 in 2000 births with a carrier rate of 1 in 20–30. There is, however, a high spontaneous mutation rate. The neonate may present with meconium ileus, requiring either a gastrografin enema or laparotomy. The cystic fibrosis gene has now been mapped to chromosome 7; however several different mutations have been discovered. Thus reliable antenatal screening can only be offered to families with a previous cystic fibrosis sufferer from whom DNA is available.

The sweat test is a useful screening test if at least 100 mg of sweat is collected. A sodium concentration of greater than 60 mmol/litre is diagnostic, and values between 40 and 60 mmol/litre necessitate a repeat examination. Other causes of a high sweat sodium concentration include Addison's disease, CAH, nephrogenic diabetes insipidus, glucose-6-phosphatase deficiency, fucosidosis and ectodermal dysplasia with hypoparathyroidism and sensorineural deafness.

Treatment of cystic fibrosis is aggressive treatment of all chest complications with physiotherapy and antibiotics and obsessional attention to nutrient intake, coupled with pancreatic replacement therapy to maintain normal height and weight velocities. However, cor pulmonale secondary to lung parenchymal damage is still a major cause of death. Heart–lung transplant is then the only option.

This child also received cereals, containing gluten, and cows' milk. Therefore, coeliac disease and cows' milk protein intolerance must be excluded. Children with coeliac disease often have a hypochromic microcytic anaemia secondary to iron deficiency but this would not be manifest at 9 months. Folate deficiency also occurs and a macrocytic blood film may occur when the iron deficiency is corrected. Diagnosis may be confirmed by duodenal or jejunal mucosal biopsy, demonstrating abnormal histology, followed by remission of symptoms when gluten is excluded from the diet.

There is a stunting or flattening of the villi and deepening of the crypts and a cellular infiltrate consisting of eosinophils and lymphocytes, with an increased number of IgM-secreting cells. These changes should revert to normal on a gluten-free diet. If the diagnosis remains in doubt after jejunal biopsy and the symptoms remain, the child should be placed on a gluten-free diet, have a repeat jejunal biopsy and then be subjected to a gluten challenge to determine the effect of gluten on the small bowel mucosa.

The diagnosis of cows' milk protein enteropathy may be difficult to substantiate. The history may be suggestive, with the onset of symptoms coinciding with the introduction of cows' milk. Jejunal mucosal damage is patchy and normal mucosa may be biopsied; double port capsules have been introduced to circumvent this problem. There are no specific histological changes in cows' milk protein enteropathy, and microscopy may reveal a non-specific partial villous atrophy. A rise in complement breakdown products following a cows' milk challenge is supportive. Recently, however, this has been questioned. Often the diagnosis is made clinically following dietary exclusion of cows' milk protein.

Lactose intolerance is commonly secondary to mucosal damage induced by gastroenteritis; primary lactose intolerance is rare. The clinical response to an oral load of lactose is of prime importance in the diagnosis; supportive evidence may be gained from a lactose tolerance test. A rise in blood glucose of less than 1.1 mmol/litre is suggestive of lactose deficiency; however, false positives can occur. Alternatively, the hydrogen breath test can be used, demonstrating a rise in end expiratory hydrogen concentration after lactose ingestion.

Decreased xylose absorption implies small bowel brush-border damage, but is of little value in differentiating the causes of an enteropathy.

Further reading

Phelan, P. D., Landau, L. I. and Olinsky, A. (eds) (1990). In *Respiratory Illness in Children*, 3rd edn, pp. 192–233. (Oxford; Blackwell Scientific Publications)

Stafford, R. J. and Grand, R. J. (1988). Diseases of the exocrine pancreas during childhood. In *Harries' Paediatric Gastroenterology*, 2nd edn, Ed. by P. J. Milla and D. P. R. Muller, pp. 369–90. (London; Churchill Livingstone)

Walker-Smith, J. A. (ed.) (1988). *Diseases of the Small Intestine*, 3rd edn, pp. 88–143. (London; Butterworths)

Case 38

Answers

1. Serum level of carbamazepine.
2. Deliberate ingestion of carbamazepine.

184

Discussion

The initial presentation of this child could suggest a migrainous episode. She had a headache, dizziness, visual disturbances and vomiting. However, the visual disturbances of migraine are usually described as flashing lights followed by bilateral scotomata; diplopia is rare, and slow pupillary reflexes are also not a feature of migraine. Ataxic gait and limb weakness may occur but the neurological symptoms usually develop rapidly and then remit equally rapidly, often within an hour, leaving the patient with a unilateral throbbing headache.

She had had a previous episode, also of short duration, some months earlier, also with no neurological sequelae. This militates against intracranial pathology, such as a space-occupying lesion or vascular accident. Central nervous system infection is similarly unlikely.

Two drugs are mentioned. Insulin overdose, with hypoglycaemic symptoms such as sweating, tachycardia, ataxia and tremor, is unlikely as she is still experiencing severe symptoms with a normal blood glucose level. The most likely diagnosis is one of carbamazepine toxicity. Carbamazepine is structurally related to the tricyclic antidepressants and its toxic effects are similar. They include headache, dizziness, drowsiness, diplopia, blurred vision, ataxia and gastrointestinal disturbance. Cardiovascular effects include hypertension, hypotension and ectopic beats. Rarer toxic effects include morbilliform skin rashes, Stevens–Johnson syndrome, bone marrow depression, jaundice and renal failure.

This child later admitted taking her father's tablets deliberately before both episodes. The psychodynamics of self-poisoning attempts are multiple and complex, but some attempts are related to specific occurrences. In this instance, the vulval bruising noted in the examination was the result of a sexual advance by the child's father.

Further reading

Baker, T. and Duncan, S. (1986). Child sexual abuse. In *Recent Advances in Paediatrics*, no. 8, Ed. by R. Meadow pp. 259–80. (Edinburgh; Churchill Livingstone)

Brett, E. (1983). *Paediatric Neurology*. Side Effects of Anticonvulsant Drugs, pp. 317–19. (Edinburgh; Churchill Livingstone)

Meadow, R. (1984). Factitious illness: the hinterland of child abuse. In *Recent Advances in Paediatrics*, no. 7, pp. 217–31. (Edinburgh; Churchill Livingstone)

Schneidman, E. S. (1975). Adolescent suicide. In *Comprehensive Textbook of Psychiatry*, 2dn edn, Ed. by A. M. Freedman, H. I. Kaplan and B. J. Sadock, p. 1774. (Baltimore; Williams & Wilkins)

Case 39

Answers

1. (a) Crohn's disease.
   (b) Tuberculous ileitis.
2. (a) Barium enema.
   (b) Colonoscopy.
   (c) Mucosal biopsy.
   (d) Mantoux test.
   (e) Chest X-ray.
   (f) Stool culture.

Discussion

The presence of a spontaneous perianal fistula, as evidenced by soiling of the underwear without incontinence, suggests Crohn's disease or, more rarely, tuberculous ileitis as possible diagnoses. Other compatible features include unaltered blood mixed with watery semi-solid stools, weight loss and a painful abdominal mass without tenesmus. Tenesmus is common in ulcerative colitis, whilst spontaneous fistulae are rare. Tuberculous enteritis and fistula-in-ano formation are rare in childhood and usually occur in children with suppurative pulmonary tuberculosis, who then swallow the infected sputum. This child had no pulmonary symptoms, but it is a diagnosis to consider in the debilitated child.

Infective causes of bloody diarrhoea such as *Shigella* and *Campylobacter* infestation should be excluded by repeated stool cultures. Intestinal mucosal infarction during a sickling crisis causes rectal bleeding. However, such episodes are accompanied by a fall in Hb level and severe abdominal pain with bleeding occurring after some days, then resolving spontaneously.

Rectal bleeding is uncommon in paediatrics and should always be investigated thoroughly. Upper intestinal bleeding, unless catastrophic, will produce malaena. Causes of frank rectal bleeding include bleeding diatheses, inflammatory bowel diseases and local causes such as rectal prolapse or fissure-in-ano. Common surgical causes are duplication cysts, volvulus and intussusception. Rarely, polyps, haemorrhoids or neoplasms may present with rectal bleeding in paediatric practice.

Further reading

Booth, I. W. and Grand, R. J. (1988). Chronic inflammatory bowel disease. In *Harries' Paediatric Gastroenterology*, 2nd edn, Ed. by P. J. Milla and D. P. R. Muller, pp. 137–69. (London; Churchill Livingstone)
Walker-Smith, J. A. (ed). (1988). Crohn's disease and abdominal tuberculosis. In *Diseases of the Small Intestine*, 3rd edn, pp. 354–8. (London; Butterworths)

Case 40

Answers

1. Inhalation of a foreign body
2. Bronchoscopy

Discussion

Inhalation of a foreign body in a child is particularly common under the age of 4 years. Peanuts and other edible nuts comprise about 50% of inhaled foreign bodies; this child inhaled a pistachio nut! The problem is fairly easy to diagnose if there is a history of inhalation followed by the onset of cough and wheeze. This is usually caused by the initial irritation following a foreign body in the airways with choking and coughing; mucosal oedema then may result from chemical irritation due to nut oils, often arachidonic acid. This may cause some wheeze, but wheeze also results from an obstructive hyperinflation of part of or all of one lung, where the foreign body acts as a ball valve allowing air in but not out. Alternatively, a collapse may occur distal to the foreign body and this can become secondarily infected.

Delay in diagnosis occurs in about a third of cases. About 40% of these are because the parents are unaware that the child has inhaled anything, as in the above case. However, attention should have been paid earlier to the fact that this girl had a cough for 3 days without a temperature or preceding coryza, followed by a severe illness with a small segmental collapse/consolidation which did not improve rapidly. Partially treated meningitis was then a complicating feature, probably from persisting septicaemia secondary to the chest infection. Hyperinflation of the left lung is an unusual feature at this stage but possibly resulted from movement of the impacted nut while coughing.

Generally the clinical picture associated with an unknown retained foreign body follows various patterns: wheeze is the most important symptom, failed resolution of an acute respiratory infection, chronic cough with haemoptysis, chronic cough and lung collapse and respiratory failure. If a child presents with a first attack of wheezy bronchitis this diagnosis should be borne in mind, but when there is a previous history of wheezing, as in this little girl, the problem is all the more difficult.

Any foreign body must be removed. Generally this is done by bronchoscopy but if the material is embedded in the bronchial wall, a segment or lobe may need to be removed. This, of course, should be preceded by a bronchoscopy. Dexamethasone and antibiotics may be necessary if the bronchoscopy is difficult.

Further reading

Dinwiddie, R. (1990). *The Diagnosis and Management of Paediatric Respiratory Disease*, pp. 223–7. (Edinburgh; Churchill Livingstone)

Rothman, B. F. *et al*. (1980). Foreign bodies in the larynx and tracheo-bronchial tree in children. A review of 225 cases. *Annals of Otology, Rhinology and Laryngology*, **89**, 434–5.

Case 41

Answers

1. (a) Toxocara indirect fluorescent antibody.
   (b) Toxocara enzyme-linked immunosorbent assay (ELISA).
   (c) Toxocara precipitin absorption.
   (d) Countercurrent immunoelectrophoresis.
   (e) Ascaris complement fixation.

2. (a) *Toxocara canis* infestation.
   (b) Ascaris species (rare).

Discussion

The most striking investigative abnormality in this child is the absolute eosinophilia. Causes of eosinophilia include allergic reactions, parasitic infestation, drugs such as penicillin and streptomycin, skin diseases (including psoriasis and pemphigus), pulmonary eosinophilia, Hodgkin's disease, eosinophilic leukaemia and polyarteritis nodosa. The length of history and lack of any systemic physical findings make malignancy unlikely and this degree of eosinophilia is particularly seen in parasitic infestations or pulmonary eosinophilia.

Pulmonary eosinophilia is classified by aetiology. Löffler's syndrome or simple pulmonary eosinophilia is probably a hypersensitivity reaction to a multitude of agents including drugs, inhaled allergens and desensitizing vaccines. Pulmonary eosinophilia occurs in a small percentage of asthmatics. The aetiology is unknown, but again may be a hypersensitivity reaction. Chest X-ray reveals patchy shadowing.

Tropical eosinophilia is similar to Löffler's syndrome but caused by the migrating larvae of filarial worms. Visceral larva migrans caused by *Toxocara canis* produces a similar syndrome in temperate climates.

The diagnosis that most closely fits with the findings in this boy of eosinophilia and an occular mass is visceral larva migrans caused by the larvae of *T. canis*. The role of *T. canis* in visceral larva migrans is still not determined.

Puppies are the main domestic carriers of *T. canis.* and there is orofaecal spread to humans. The soil in many parklands and waste areas contains viable toxocara eggs which can be ingested by children. The eggs hatch in the intestine and the larvae migrate randomly through the body and may encyst in any organ. The younger child usually has systemic signs and symptoms such as pyrexia, pica, failure to thrive, anaemia and hepatosplenomegaly. Involvement of the lung produces cough and wheezing. Neurological involvement may cause bizarre peripheral signs, fits or coma. In the older child it is not uncommon for the eye alone to be affected, with no other physical findings. Asymptomatic siblings of affected children are occasionally shown to have hepatomegaly and eosinophilia. Certain diagnosis can be gained only by biopsy, but the indirect fluorescent antibody test and toxocara skin test are becoming more reliable. Both serology and skin test may be negative if the infection is confined to the eye. Treatment of visceral larva migrans is with diethylcarbamazine or thiobendazole.

The larvae of certain other worms are capable of causing visceral larva migrans. Such worms include *Ascaris suum* from pigs and, rarely, *A. lumbricoides*. Again, intense eosinophilia is seen, but it is extremely rare to have a single ocular granulomatous lesion with no other manifestations.

Further reading

Lynch, N. R., Wilkes, L. K., Hodgen, A. N. and Turner, K. J. (1988). Specificity of toxocara ELISA in tropical populations. *Parasite Immunology*, **10**, 323–37.

Safar, E. H., Azab, M. E., Khalil, H. M., Bebars, M. A., el Hady, H. and Khattab, H. M. (1990). Immunodiagnostics of *Toxocara canis* in suspected ocular and visceral manifestations. *Folia Parasitologica*, **37**, 249–54.

Case 42

Answers

1. Fanconi syndrome.
2. Cystinosis.
3. (a) Urinary amino acids.
   (b) Slit lamp examination of the eye.
   (c) Bone marrow aspiration.
   (d) Lymph node biopsy.
   (e) Sodium bicarbonate loading either by infusion or orally.
   (f) Urinary phosphate excretion.
   (g) Urinary potassium.
4. (a) Potassium supplementation.
   (b) Correction of acidosis with citrate solution and/or sodium bicarbonate.
   (c) Vitamin D supplements or an analogue such as 1 α-hydroxycholecalciferol.
   (d) Sufficient fluid intake.
   (e) Hydrochlorothiazide.

5. (a) Complicating an inborn error of metabolism, i.e. tyrosinae-
mia; hereditary fructose intolerance; Wilson's disease; galactosaemia; glycogen storage disease.
   (b) Lowe's syndrome (oculocerebral renal syndrome).
   (c) Idiopathic.
   (d) Heavy metal poisoning, e.g. lead.

Discussion

This child presents a classic picture of Fanconi syndrome: a
normal child at birth developing growth failure with rickets,
constipation and finally an acute illness secondary to renal pathology. Fanconi syndrome consists of renal tubular acidosis affecting the proximal tubules, together with generalized aminoaciduria, glycosuria, hyperphosphaturia and hypokalaemia.

In proximal renal tubular acidosis (PTA) there is reduced
reabsorption of bicarbonate even with a mild acidosis present, in
effect a lowered bicarbonate threshold. Below this bicarbonate
level there are sufficient hydrogen ions secreted by the proximal
tubule to reabsorb bicarbonate. Distal tubular function is intact,
thus in a case such as this the urinary pH is appropriately acidic,
unlike distal tubular acidosis where an alkaline urine is found
despite a metabolic acidosis.

In normal patients the bicarbonate renal threshold is
24–26 mmol/litre. Sodium bicarbonate supplements in the order
of 5–15 mmol/kg/24 hours can be given in PTA for maintenance
but generally a mixture of sodium and potassium citrate is given
to correct the acidosis and electrolyte deficit.

Potassium is lost from both proximal and distal tubules, resulting in severe weakness, thus large amounts of potassium, usually
in the citrate mixture as described above, are given as maintenance once the initial deficit has been corrected. Hypokalaemia
plus tubular damage occurring as a result of the primary pathology can impair the ability to concentrate the urine. Thus diarrhoea and vomiting result in very rapid dehydration and acidosis. These episodes can cause episodic fever.

Hyperphosphaturia results in hypophosphataemia initially.
Sometimes phosphate supplements are required, and only as
renal function fails does the serum phosphate level rise. Hyper-
calciuria occurs but secondary hyperparathyroidism maintains a
normal serum calcium at the expense of the bones, which become demineralized causing rickets or osteomalacia. Vitamin D is

given but there is resistance to several of the effects. However, large doses may improve calcium absorption and partially restore tubular transport of amino acids, glucose and phosphate. Intestinal absorption of calcium is not always depressed in multiple tubular dysfunction; thus calcium supplements are only sometimes required. The vitamin D analogue 1 α-hydroxycholecalciferol is an easier medication to use since it bypasses the kidney hydroxylation of vitamin D to its active metabolite, 1,25-dihydroxycholecalciferol, and has a short half-life.

Cystinosis is the most likely diagnosis since the parents were first cousins and the family history is in favour of an autosomal recessive inheritance. Cystine crystals are most readily demonstrated in the cornea by slit lamp examination, also in bone marrow aspirates. At a later stage the cornea becomes cloudy. Deposits are also found in the rest of the reticuloendothelial system, i.e. liver, spleen and lymph nodes, and may be seen in biopsy material.

Hydrochlorothiazide given for maintenance therapy may facilitate the correction of acidosis and healing of rickets by increasing proximal tubular absorption of sodium, bicarbonate, phosphate and calcium. In turn this should reduce the solute load in the urine and thus the degree of polyuria. Fluid intake must always be great enough to balance the obligatory polyuria.

Further reading

Brodehl, J. (1978). The Fanconi syndrome. In *Paediatric Kidney Disease*, Ed. by C. N. Edelmann, p. 81. (Boston; Little, Brown)

Pennock, C. A. (1987). Lysosomal storage disorders, In *Inherited Metabolic Diseases*, Ed. by J. B. Holton, pp. 91–2. (Edinburgh; Churchill Livingstone)

Postlethwaite, R. J. (1986). Renal tubular disorders. In *Clinical Paediatric Nephrology*, Ed. by R. J. Postlethwaite, pp. 238–48. (Bristol; Wright)

Case 43

Answers

1. Acute intermittent porphyria.
2. Autosomal dominant.

Discussion

The behaviour of the child after parental separation had been appropriate, if unreasonable. However, there had been a recent behavioural change with inappropriate responses, usually associated with abdominal pain. During one such attack–probably precipitated by otitis media–hyponatraemia, leukocytosis, hypertension, pigmentation and a loss of deep tendon reflexes were observed. These findings are consistent with acute intermittent porphyria. Porphyria variegata differs clinically in the skin manifestations which include a photosensitive rash with blistering and cicatrization. Temporal lobe epilepsy had been excluded by an EEG and a trial of carbamazepine. Many aspects of this case are seen in chronic lead intoxication, but not hyponatraemia, uraemia, a normal Hb level and pigmentation. The recurrent nature of the episodes is also not characteristic.

Porphyria is a rare disease, subdivided into three groups: erythropoietic, erythrohepatic and hepatic. Acute intermittent porphyria and porphyria variegata are hepatic variants. Inheritance of both is autosomal dominant and attacks, which may last from hours to weeks, occur after puberty, more commonly in females. Episodes may be precipitated by drugs such as barbiturates, sulphonamides and griseofulvin, hormones such as oestrogens, infection and dieting. Abdominal symptoms include localized or generalized pain variably accompanied by vomiting and constipation; neurological symptoms are more varied and range from personality changes and mild neurological deficits to quadriplegia and death from respiratory paralysis. Skin manifestations are usually confined to pigmentation without blistering in areas exposed to sunlight. Biochemical abnormalities include hyponatraemia and uraemia, and less commonly hypokalaemia and hypochloraemia.

Diagnosis is confirmed by detecting elevated levels of porphyrin precursors in the urine and faeces. In acute intermittent porphyria δ-aminolevulinic acid and porphobilinogen are markedly increased in the urine and coproporphyrinogen and uroporphyrinogen in the faeces are either normal or slightly increased. In porphyria variegata, the urinary findings are similar but there is a marked increase in faecal porphyrins. Lead poisoning can be differentiated by a normal porphobilinogen and raised δ-aminolevulinic acid level.

Erythrocyte levels of uroporphyrinogen-1-synthetase may be reduced in acute intermittent porphyria but this is an unreliable indication.

Urinary coproporphyrinogen may be increased in liver disease; ulcerative lesions of upper gastrointestinal tract may produce increased faecal porphyrins from denaturation of Hb.

Treatment is by avoiding precipitating factors as far as possible and correcting electrolyte imbalance during the episode.

Further reading

Bissell, D. M. and Schmid, R. (1982). Hepatic porphyrias. In *Diseases of the Liver*, 5th edn, Ed. by L. Schiff and E. R. Schiff. (Philadelphia; J. P. Lippincott)

Boon, F. F. and Ellis, C. (1989). Acute intermittent porphyria in a children's psychiatric hospital. *Journal of the American Academy of Child and Adolescent Psychiatry*, **28**, 606–9.

McNeely, M. D. D. (1980). Liver function. In *Gradwohl's Clinical Laboratory Methods and Diagnosis*, 8th edn, Ed. by A. C. Sonnenwirth and L. J. Jarett, pp. 548–50 (St. Louis; C. V. Mosby)

Case 44

Answers

1. (a) Pyloric stenosis.
   (b) Hiatus hernia or gastro-oesophageal reflux.
   (c) Cows' milk intolerance.
   (d) Inborn error of metabolism: organic aciduria.
   (e) Raised intracranial pressure.
2. (a) Test feed.
   (b) Barium swallow and follow-through, or ultrasound.
   (c) pH and calculation of anion gap (the difference between the sum of cation concentration, i.e. Na^+ and K^+, and that of anions, i.e. Cl^- and HCO_3^-)
   (d) Urinary and plasma amino acid profile.
   (e) Blood ammonia.
   (f) Blood lactic acid level.
   (g) Jejunal biopsy.
   (h) Radioallergosorbent test–specific IgE for cows milk.
   (i) CT scan.

Discussion

This child presents with a classic history of pyloric stenosis, in a form not seen so frequently today. Pyloric stenosis should always be considered in a previously healthy baby, particularly a boy, aged 1–3 months, who has significant vomiting. Five times as many cases occur in male than in female infants. The onset often occurs in the second or third week with non-projectile vomiting, which proceeds to projectile vomiting, either after every feed or intermittently. The infant is usually hungry and is anxious to take another feed immediately. Sometimes the baby becomes lethargic, as in this case, and only small volumes of feed are taken. With such poor intake and incomplete pyloric obstruction, little or no vomiting occurs, but there is marked failure to thrive. Full-volume tube feeds will result in increased vomiting and visible gastric peristalsis. Typically there is hypochloroaemic alkalosis, variable dehydration, and sodium and potassium losses.

To try to prove pyloric stenosis a test feed is generally given, first to see gastric peristalsis and secondly to feel the pyloric tumour. A barium meal can be carried out if the test feed is inconclusive. This will show delayed gastric emptying and the 'string sign' of the narrow elongated pyloric canal and a 'mushroom' effect of the duodenal cap. Ultrasound has recently been used to demonstrate the pyloric mass.

Differential diagnoses of cows' milk intolerance, hiatus hernia or gastro-oesophageal reflux are possible. Hiatus hernia and gastro-oesophageal reflux do not generally cause marked metabolic abnormalities; reluctance to feed is very unusual, but failure to thrive is common; there may be iron-deficiency anaemia from bleeding in hiatus hernia. Diagnosis should be by barium swallow, or oesophageal pH monitoring if this is available.

Cows' milk intolerance often presents with a history of reluctance to take feeds and vomiting, but frequently there are other symptoms such as diarrhoea, irritability, rash, wheezing and blood in the stools–not present in this case. A jejunal biopsy should show a non-specific small bowel enteropathy. Serial biopsies following a milk-free diet and subsequent cows' milk challenge are the best method of diagnosis. Specific IgE for cows' milk does not correspond well with clinical status.

This history is suggestive of an inborn error of metabolism, many of which are associated with an unexplained acidosis. This is significant if the anion gap exceeds 16 mmol/litre, when abnormal levels of ketones, lactate or organic acids should be sought. Proprionic acidaemia and methylmalonic acidaemia, examples of organic acidurias, usually present with disease early in life, but occasionally presentation is delayed up to the age of 3 months. Failure to thrive, with vomiting and marked intolerance to the usual dietary intake of protein, are the presenting symptoms. There can also be episodes of acute illness heralded by keto-nuria. This is followed by vomiting which may be so severe that it suggests the presence of pyloric stenosis. Hyperammonaemia can be found in both organic acidurias and with defects of the enzymes of the urea cycle. In the latter, progressive lethargy commonly develops within the first 48 hours of life. This may be associated with jerky movements or frank seizures, before progressing to deep coma. This case has many clinical features of the delayed-type presentation of methylmalonic acidaemia but the raised HCO_3^- value suggests alkalosis rather than acidosis. Lactic acidosis as a result of disorders of the pyruvate dehy-drogenase complex, is unlikely for the same reason, and most cases have marked signs by the age of 3 months. Hyperglycinae-mia may present with episodes of ketonuria, hypoglycaemia, vomiting, fits etc.; raised plasma amino acids and aminoaciduria may be found.

Inborn errors of carbohydrate metabolism are unlikely to pre-sent at the age of 2–3 months. Reducing substances should be present in the urine, and clinical features of hepatomegaly, jaundice, cataracts, irritability and convulsions may be marked at this stage.

Lastly, alteration of behaviour with vomiting and lethargy should always suggest an intracranial lesion. A CT scan should assist diagnosis.

Further reading

Chalmer, R. A. (1987). Disorders of organic acid metabolism. In *The Inherited Metabolic Disease*, Ed. by J. B. Holton, pp. 141–211. (Edinburgh; Churchill Livingstone)

Milla, P. J. and Muller, D. P. R. (1988). *Harries' Paediatric Gastroenterology*, 2nd edn, pp. 86–8, 119–22, 197–9 (London; Churchill Livingstone)

Nixon, H. and O'Donnell, B. (1992). *Essentials of Paediatric Surgery*. 4th Edn. (Oxford; Butterworth-Heinemann)

Pollitt, R. J. (1987). Amino acid disorders. In *The Inherited Metabolic Disease*, Ed. by J. B. Holton, pp. 96–139 (Edinburgh; Churchill Livingstone)

Case 45

Answers

1. (a) Galactosaemia.
   (b) Fructosaemia.
   (c) Neonatal hepatitis.
   (d) Sepsis.
2. (a) Conjugated and unconjugated bilirubin.
   (b) Blood cultures.
   (c) Analysis of the reducing substance.
   (d) Urinalysis for protein and amino acids.
   (e) Enzyme levels.

Discussion

The presenting clinical sign in this child is prolonged jaundice, the causes of which are protean. It is diagnostically useful, therefore, to determine the relative amounts of conjugated and unconjugated bilirubin. Further positive signs are vomiting with non-bloody diarrhoea, hepatomegaly and poor weight gain. Positive laboratory data include hypoglycaemia, with reducing substances in the urine, prolonged PTT/KCT, and a metabolic acidosis associated with a neutral urinary pH, suggesting a tubular defect in hydrogen homeostasis. Those features are compatible with galactosaemia and fructosaemia; the infant must have previously ingested the relevant sugar. However, some other diagnoses to exclude are neonatal hepatitis, sepsis and Fanconi's syndrome. Neonatal hepatitis, unlike cirrhosis, is not associated with renal abnormalities, but it may be associated with hypoglycaemia secondary to the compromised liver. Galactosuria may occur as the insulted liver is unable to metabolize galactose rapidly, resulting in urinary excretion.

Sepsis may cause hypoglycaemia, a metabolic acidosis, which is combined with an acid urine and unconjugated hyperbilirubinaemia. It is not associated with galactosuria but should, nevertheless, be excluded. Fanconi's syndrome, which produces renal tubular acidosis, is not associated with jaundice, and hypoglycaemia is rare, despite glycosuria.

Galactosaemia is a rare, recessively inherited disease occurring in between 1 in 30 000 to 1 in 70 000 live births. Two types occur related to different enzyme defects. Galactokinase deficiency is associated with cataract formation only; galactose-1-phosphate uridyl transferase deficiency causes multi-system involvement of widely varying severity. The mild Duarte variant causes no symptoms but erythrocyte galactose-1-phosphate uridyl transferase activity is reduced. The more severe forms present a few days after the ingestion of lactose.

Prolonged jaundice is often the presenting sign. Diarrhoea and vomiting, hepatomegaly and failure to thrive follow rapidly. Cataracts may occur in the first few days of life, but are visible with a slit lamp only as they consist of small punctate lesions in the fetal lens nucleus. Hypoglycaemia, secondary to galactose ingestion, is caused by the inhibition of phosphoglucomutase and glucose-6-phosphatase by galactose-1-phosphate. Hepatic damage causes hepatomegaly, jaundice, hypoproteinaemia and hypoprothrombinaemia. Early biopsy reveals fatty infiltration, fibrosis, bile duct proliferation and a characteristic pseudoalveolar arrangement of hepatic cells. Later macronodular cirrhosis supervenes. Renal accumulation of galactose-1-phosphate induces proximal tubular acidosis, phosphaturia, bicarbonaturia producing acidosis, proteinuria and generalized aminoaciduria. The aminoaciduria is non-specific, but there is a predominance of the neutral dibasic acids serine, glycine, alanine, threonine, glutamine and valine. The phosphaturia may cause rickets. Rarely, pseudotumor cerebri occurs secondary to diffuse cerebral oedema.

Treatment consists of a lactose-free diet, for example Nutramigen. Therapeutic efficacy is followed by serial measurements of erythrocyte galactose-1-phosphate level.

Fructosaemia is an equally rare autosomal recessively inherited disease with an incidence of approximately 1 in 40 000 live births. Two varieties occur: fructokinase deficiency which causes benign fructosuria only, and the more severe fructose-1-phosphate aldolase deficiency with accumulation of fructose-1-phosphate in many tissues, which causes widespread systemic effects.

There are three aldolase isoenzymes: A in muscle, B in liver and C in the brain; in this disease the liver isoenzyme is deficient.

Clinical presentation of fructose-1-phosphate aldolase deficiency varies with age. In the infant, severe hypoglycaemia is induced 20–30 min after ingestion of fructose, accompanied by sweating, irritability, vomiting and possibly convulsions with loss of consciousness. If the diagnosis is missed, chronic fructose poisoning causes jaundice, fatty infiltration of the liver, hepatomegaly and hepatocyte cytoplasmic dissolution; eventually cirrhosis supervenes with ascites and oedema. The vomiting worsens in frequency and severity and the child fails to thrive. Accumulation of fructose-1-phosphate in the kidney produces a proximal tubular acidosis, phosphaturia, proteinuria and aminoaciduria.

In the older child, hypoglycaemia is normally not a feature, but shortly after ingestion of fructose severe epigastric pain is experienced, followed by nausea and vomiting.

Diagnosis is confirmed by detecting fructosaemia, hyperbilirubinaemia, hypophosphataemia, raised free fatty acids and raised liver enzymes. Fructosuria, phosphaturia, proteinuria and aminoaciduria occur. Fructose tolerance tests should be performed with extreme care, if at all, as profound hypoglycaemia, sufficient to cause neurological damage, may occur.

Treatment is a fructose-free diet and the prognosis is generally good; however, a more guarded opinion must be given in the more severe cases.

Further reading

Baerlocher, K., Gitzelman, R. G. and Steinmann, B. (1980). Disorders in fructose metabolism. In *Inherited Disorders of Carbohydrate Metabolism*, Ed. by D. Burman, J. B. Holton and C. A. Pennod, pp. 165–75. (London; MTP Press)

Gitzelman, R. and Hansen, R. G. (1980). Galactose metabolism, hereditary defects and their clinical significance. In *Inherited Disorders of Carbohydrate Metabolism*, Ed. by D. Burman, J. B. Holton and C. A. Pennod, pp. 71–94. (London; MTP Press)

Case 46

Answers

1. (a) Dermatomyositis.
   (b) Polymyostis.
   (c) Limb girdle muscular dystrophy.
   (d) Viral infection with myositis.
2. (a) Creatine kinase.
   (b) Electromyogram (EMG).
   (c) Muscle biopsy.
   (d) Muscle ultrasound imaging.
   (e) Viral studies.
   (f) Bone marrow aspiration.
3. (a) Collodion patches (erythematous scaly patches).
   (b) Calcinotic nodules/subcutaneous calcification.
   (c) Telangiectasia on eyelids and nailbeds.

(d) Retinitis.
(e) Palatorespiratory muscle involvement leading to respiratory difficulties and aspiration.
(f) Dysphagia.
(g) Haematemesis and melaena from ulceration.

Discussion

Dermatomyositis is usually diagnosed on the clinical features of polymyositis and typical skin rashes, and confirmed by elevation of creatine kinase, an abnormal EMG and muscle biopsy samples showing inflammatory myositis. Dermatomyositis in childhood has been recorded in association with leukaemia and hypogamma-globulinaemia, but this is rare. In adults there is a 20% association with malignancy. Connective tissue diseases are also found in association in all age groups. The most prominent pathological process in children is a vasculitis involving arterioles, venules and capillaries in connective tissues of the skin, subcutaneous tissue and muscle. This accounts for the characteristic lesions seen. Onset is usually subacute following a viral infection but may be insidious with weakness of the proximal leg muscles and also sometimes the shoulder girdle muscles. This is often asymmetrical, but when symmetric can mimic limb girdle muscular dystrophy. Distal muscles may also be involved, particularly the calf muscles, presenting with contractures and toe-walking. Pain and tenderness in the muscles may be prominent and difficult to distinguish from joint pain. The anterior neck muscles are often affected causing weakness of neck flexion.

The above case exhibits only some of the other typical features with fever, pain, weight loss, general malaise, non-pitting oedema and typical facial rash, especially in the periorbital and malar areas. The rash may extend to the neck, shoulders, upper chest, extensor surfaces and front of legs. There may be red patches over bony prominences, such as the knuckles, which can flake and are then called collodion patches; telangiectasia around the nail beds; calcium is deposited in the skin and subcutaneous tissues in 50% of cases, forming sheets or nodules which may extrude–this is very rare in adults; mucous membrane involvement with dysphagia is mainly seen in adults; retinitis with 'cotton-wool' exudates; and acute respiratory difficulties.

The clinical picture should make the diagnosis here. Limb girdle muscular dystrophy is unlikely in view of the rapid onset, constitutional upset, rash and muscle tenderness. Creatine kinase would probably be raised in all three conditions, but EMG should show myopathic features in limb girdle muscular dystrophy, whereas fibrillation potentials are also present in polymyositis and dermatomyositis, similar to those seen in denervating disorders. Muscle biopsy should distinguish between those two. Recently muscle ultrasound has proved a useful screening technique for muscle pathology.

Other differential diagnoses are transient myositis following a viral infection such as influenza; trichinosis, which presents with muscle tenderness and eosinophilia; Guillain–Barré syndrome; also connective tissue disorders such as juvenile rheumatoid arthritis and scleroderma, in which varying degrees of myositis occur. Finally bone marrow aspiration should always be done in a known leukaemic patient who presents with aches and pains in the limbs.

Further reading

Brett, E. (1991). *Paediatric Neurology*, pp. 55–71, 87–90. (Edinburgh; Churchill Livingstone)

Cassidy, J. T. and Petty, R. E. (1990). *Textbook of Paediatric Rheumatology*, 2nd edn, pp. 331–67, 482–3. (New York; Churchill Livingstone)

Dubowitz, V. (1989). *A Colour Atlas of Muscle Disorders in Childhood*, pp. 158–76. (London; Wolfe)

Case 47

Answers

1. (a) Astrocytoma.
   (b) Medulloblastoma.
2. (a) MRI scan.
   (b) CT scan.

Discussion

This girl has signs of raised intracranial pressure: headache with vomiting, papilloedema, raised blood pressure and erosion of the posterior clinoid process on skull X-ray. There are innumerable causes of raised intracranial pressure, but examination revealed a truncal ataxia, which suggests a lesion in the vermis of the cerebellum. The unsteady gait is also a feature of cerebellar space-occupying lesions. The most likely lesion is a tumour, either an astrocytoma or a medulloblastoma. Hydrocephalus producing raised intracranial pressure is produced early as the aqueduct is compromised, so signs of raised intracranial pressure may occur before localizing signs.

Medulloblastomas have a peak incidence between 1 and 5 years, are rapid-growing and, therefore, present after a short history.

Astrocytomas have a peak incidence between 5 and 10 years, are slow-growing and present after a longer history. This is, therefore, the most likely diagnosis in this child.

Astrocytomas are usually benign lesions causing symptoms by slow growth, often with cyst formation. They may arise in the cerebellum, brainstem, third ventricle or cerebrum; the cerebellum is the commonest site.

The presenting signs of a cerebellar lesion are usually those of raised intracranial pressure with cerebellar signs developing subsequently. The history may be punctuated by periods of remission or conversely by rapid deterioration caused by a sudden increase in intracranial pressure by cysts blocking the ventricular system.

Brainstem astrocytomas tend to be more diffuse so surgery is only indicated for decompression and radiotherapy is the treatment of choice. There is a classic triad of symptoms, comprising multiple cranial nerve lesions, ataxia and pyramidal abnormalities. Signs of raised intracranial pressure tend to occur late.

Third ventricle astrocytomas may present with hypothalamic dysfunction and visual loss from destruction of the surrounding structures and pressure on the optic chiasma. A lesion in the anterior wall of the third ventricle may produce the diencephalic syndrome of infancy. This syndrome often presents around 6 months of age with vomiting and extreme emaciation despite adequate calorie intake. Other features include sweating, hypoglycaemia, optic atrophy, nystagmus and a 'defiantly cheerful' demeanour.

Cerebral astrocytomas are rare in childhood and present with convulsions or signs of raised intracranial pressure after reaching a considerable size.

Medulloblastomas arise in the cerebellar vermis and expand rapidly into the fourth ventricle and cerebellar hemispheres, causing cerebellar signs early in the history. Once the tumour is in the fourth ventricle, seeding may occur throughout the ventricular system. Seeding may also occur into the subarachnoid space, producing a malignant meningitis and allowing the possibility of seeding in the spinal column, causing such signs as backache, lower limb weakness and bladder dysfunction. Distant metastases are rare and usually occur in the bone marrow. Treatment is by surgical excision and decompression of the hydrocephalus if necessary, followed by combined radiotherapy and chemotherapy.

Further reading

Finlay, J. L. and Goins, S. C. (1987). Brain tumors in children. I. Advances in diagnosis. *American Journal of Pediatric Hematology-Oncology*, **9**, 246–55.

Finlay, J. L. and Goins, S. C. (1987). Brain tumors in children. III. Advances in chemotherapy. *American Journal of Pediatric Hematology-Oncology*, **9**, 264–71.

Finlay, J. L., Uteg, R. and Giese, W. L. (1987). Brain tumors in children. II. Advances in neurosurgery and radiation. *American Journal of Pediatric Hematology-Oncology*, **9**, 256–63.

Case 48

Answers

1. (a) Lateral skull X-ray for intracerebral calcification.
   (b) Toxoplasma indirect fluorescent antibody titre.
   (c) Toxoplasma antigen.
   (d) CMV-specific IgM.
2. (a) Congenital *Toxoplasma gondii* infection.
   (b) Congenital CMV infection.
   (c) Congenital herpes hominis infection.

Discussion

The most likely cause of this child's neonatal problems is an intrauterine infection producing a week-long rash and prolonged jaundice. Microcephaly is commoner than hydrocephalus in congenital rubella, so the most likely infecting agents are CMV and toxoplasmosis. These would also explain the choroidoretinitis. A lateral skull X-ray may demonstrate intracerebral calcification. Classically this should be periventricular in CMV and diffuse in toxoplasmosis. Rarely, disseminated congenital herpes hominis infection causes intracranial calcification.

Toxoplasma gondii is a ubiquitous obligate intracellular parasite. The mode of spread is unclear; certainly this protozoon is rampant both in wild and in domestic animals. Uncooked meats may, therefore, be a source. The only animal found to pass infected faeces is the cat. Once infection occurs many organs are affected, which explains the diversity of the disease manifestations.

The congenitally acquired infection, transmitted transplacentally, may cause widespread cellular damage. The commonest sign is choroidoretinitis, which affects both macular and peripheral areas. Other features include convulsions, intracranial calcification hydrocephalus, anaemia, a petechial or maculopapular rash, prolonged neonatal jaundice, hepatosplenomegaly and an abnormal CSF. The CSF may be xanthochromic and display a leukocytosis, predominantly mononuclear; the protein may be raised to levels of up to 20 g/litre.

The neurological damage is usually the most devastating, although the organism is disseminated throughout the body. Meningoencephalomyelitis occurs, with large inflammatory lesions containing necrotic centres.

Eventually calcification and cyst formation occur. Areas involved are the cortex, subcortical white matter, caudate and lenticulate nuclei, midbrain, pons, medulla oblongata and spinal cord. Hydrocephalus is caused by obstruction of the foramina of Munro or the aqueduct of Sylvius.

Fetal infection may cause a severe, rapidly fatal infection; however, less than 40% of infants born to infected mothers are themselves infected, and of those only 11% have overt disease.

Initially the toxoplasma dye test is positive and there is an increase in the indirect fluorescent antibody titre. Complement-fixing antibodies are absent initially but later rise to high levels. Toxoplasma antigen can now be detected and is used to facilitate early diagnosis. Maternal antibodies may cross the placenta and cause a high antibody titre in an uninfected infant. The titre will gradually fall over the first 4 months of life; in the infected infant the titre rises. The toxoplasma indirect fluorescent antibody titre will be raised in this child.

CMV, a DNA virus, is also widespread. Neonatal infection may be transplacental or via contact with infected cervical secretions.

Only the minority of infants born to infected mothers have overt disease, which may range from mild and self-limiting to fatal.

A diffuse petechial rash may occur within a few hours or days postnatally, secondary to thrombocytopenia, which usually clears rapidly, but the hepatitis-induced jaundice may persist for up to 4 months. Neurological abnormalities include choroidoretinitis, spasticity, convulsions, microcephaly, hydrocephalus and cerebral calcification, usually periventricular. However, all major systems are involved causing cardiac, gastrointestinal and musculoskeletal abnormalities.

'Owl eye' cells, caused by intranuclear inclusion bodies, may be seen in the urine or the virus may be cultured in tissue culture. Immunological markers are the neutralizing antibody, indirect fluorescent antibody or complement fixation tests. The most rapid neonatal test is the detection of a raised CMV IgM titre, which is positive for several years.

Further reading

Kinney, J. S. and Kumar, M. L. (1988). Should we expand the TORCH complex? A description of clinical and diagnostic aspects of selected old and new agents. *Clinics in Perinatology*, **15**, 727–44.

Krugman, S., Katz, S. L., Gershon, A. A. and Wilfert, C. (eds) (1991). *Infectious Diseases of Children*, 9th edn., pp. 25–41, 518–48. (London; C. V. Mosby)

Case 49

Answers

1. (a) The family history of migraine.
   (b) Associated symptoms of attacks, i.e. visual, headache, giddiness, motor, sensory, seizures and autonomic symptoms.
2. (a) EEG.
   (b) Therapeutic trial of ergotamine, propranolol or pizotifen.

Discussion

The diagnosis here is migraine, but of a variant type. Differentiation from the partial seizure form of epilepsy can sometimes be difficult. All types of migraine occur in children: classic or common, in which an aura does not precede the headache; cluster headaches; hemiplegic; opththalmoplegic and basilar artery migraine. Children with migraine equivalents may pose difficult problems in diagnosis. The most common is the recurrent abdominal syndrome in which there is recurrent abdominal pain with or without nausea, vomiting, cyclic vomiting, fever, chest pain, leg cramps and autonomic symptoms such as sweating, pallor, nasal congestion and eye watering. Headache, giddiness, photophobia and a confusional state with the child 'not quite himself' may also be present, but a good history can be notoriously difficult to obtain from a young child and his parents. A family history of migraine is present in a majority of children presenting with migraine.

Pointers to this child having migraine are the sudden cessation of pain and vomiting after comparatively long episodes lasting 24 hours and lack of any type of obvious seizures. There is an interesting relationship between epilepsy and migraine, the subject of much debate since one follows the other at times. Epileptic attacks may involve abdominal pain or headache, migraine attacks may occasionally be associated with loss of consciousness or convulsion probably due to syncope. EEG abnormalities occur in about 20% of patients with recurrent abdominal syndrome, but on follow-up some years later most patients are symptom-free. There is a sizeable amount of literature on the various abnormalities found in the EEG of migrainous patients. Great care must be taken in its interpretation; an accurate history is still the cornerstone to diagnosis.

Migraine can be precipitated by a number of triggers, i.e. dietary, stress, anxiety, tiredness. These must be addressed as in recurrent abdominal pain in childhood. Often once the anxiety that something is 'seriously wrong' has been taken away, the situation may improve spontaneously.

There are no definite diagnostic procedures available, but a therapeutic trial of oral ergotamine may be tried early in the course of an attack. Propranolol or the serotonin antagonist pizotifen can be used prophylactically in migraine and are effective in a number of children. Anticonvulsants may reduce the number of migraine attacks as well as epileptic episodes, but are not recommended–neither are antidepressants which have at times been used with some effect in migraine, since the number of attacks increases with depression. This was thought to be a factor in this child by his general practitioner because of the decrease

206

in attention from his mother due to illness in the fostered boy. This turned out not to be the case.

Porphyria should be considered in the differential diagnosis of abdominal pain in a child, even though it is rare. The family history, possible precipitating factors and associated symptoms should be sought. Presentation with abdominal pain, vomiting, neuropsychiatric symptoms and finally muscular weakness or paralysis can make it very similar to migraine initially. Visual disturbances and convulsions occur late. On examination there is often marked tachycardia, hypertension and neurological abnormalities. In this case the diagnosis is unlikely in view of the normal urinary porphobilinogen result, although there are some very rare forms of porphyria in which this is raised only during an attack.

Further reading

Aicardi, J. (1985). Epileptic syndromes in childhood: overview and classification. In *Paediatric Perspectives on Epilepsy*, Ed. by E. Ross and R. Reynolds. pp 65–71. (Chichester; John Wiley and Sons)

Barlow, C. F. (1984). Headaches and migraine in childhood. *Spastics International Medical Publications* (London; Blackwell Scientific)

Brett, E. M. (1991). *Paediatric Neurology*, pp. 556–63. (Edinburgh; Churchill Livingstone)

Fenichel, G. M. (1985). Migraine in children. In *Neurologic Clinics of North America vol. 3:1: Paediatric Neurology*, pp. 77–94. (Philadelphia; W. B. Saunders)

Fenton, T. R. and Milla, P. J. (1988). Recurrent abdominal pain. In *Harries' Paediatric Gastroenterology*, Ed. by P. J. Milla and D. P. R. Muller, pp. 272–6. (London; Churchill Livingstone)

Case 50

Answers

1. (a) Wilson's disease.
   (b) Chronic active hepatitis.
   (c) Halothane hepatitis.
   (d) Hepatitis C (non-A, non-B hepatitis).
   (e) α_1-Antitrypsin deficiency.
   (f) Other toxic injury–drugs, chemicals, plants.

2. (a) Serum ceruloplasmin.
   (b) Urinary copper excretion before and after penicillamine.
   (c) Slit lamp examination for Kayser–Fleischer rings.
   (d) Hepatitis C antibodies.
   (e) Halothane antibodies.
   (f) Liver scan.
   (g) Protein electrophoretic strip.
   (h) α_1-Antitrypsin protease inhibitor phenotype.
   (i) HLA type.
3. (a) Vitamin K.
   (b) Fresh frozen plasma.
   (c) Gut antibiotics, i.e. neomycin.
   (d) Lactulose.
   (e) Low-protein diet and vitamin supplementation.
   (f) Histamine H_2 receptor antagonist.
   (g) Monitor and correct any fluid/electrolyte imbalance.

Discussion

The 8-year-old boy has symptoms, signs and laboratory investigations consistent with a chronic hepatitic pathology, i.e. symptoms persisting over a period longer than 8 weeks: normal-size but non-tender liver, rising conjugated hyperbilirubinaemia, low albumin and very prolonged clotting studies. The raised ammonia and deteriorating liver function together with the vomiting, abdominal pain, headache and intermittent behavioural difficulties, suggest early hepatic encephalopathy. On looking back through the history, this boy had multiple anaesthetics, some given within 24 hours of each other. There appears to be a temporal relationship between his symptoms and the anaesthetics, starting 10 days afterwards but reducing to 5 days on the third admission. It is possible there could be two pathologies–an underlying chronic hepatitis with an overlying secondary stress causing the acute episodes.

The possible diagnosis in this child range over a wide spectrum. The first impression is of an acute hepatitis with a high IgM, then rising IgG, but both hepatitis B surface antigen (HBS Ag) and hepatitis A virus (HAV) IgM were negative. Hepatitis C is a possibility but there is no history of previous blood transfusion, and this is thought to be a method of transmission. Recently a serological test for hepatitis C antibodies has been developed. It is only positive after 3–4 months and the specificity is not yet known.

The most important diagnosis to rule out is Wilson's disease because it can present in both acute and chronic form, and is eminently treatable, with favourable outcome if diagnosis is made early. Non-hepatitic presentations in Wilson's disease can be with neurological disorders, particularly co-ordination and behavioural problems; slurring of speech; renal disorders with mild to heavy proteinuria and generalized aminoaciduria; there may be a Fanconi-type syndrome with rickets; abdominal pain; acute haemolysis, fever and arthralgia. Diagnosis is by low serum ceruloplasmin and raised urinary copper estimations, also slit lamp examination to look for Kayser–Fleischer rings in the eyes.

Autoimmune chronic active hepatitis (ACAH) is characterized by chronic aggressive hepatitis with or without cirrhosis, high concentrations of serum immunoglobulins and the presence of non-organ-specific autoantibodies in the absence of other causes of liver disease. ACAH should be treated early with immunosuppressive agents, which have been shown to improve prognosis; therefore diagnosis is important and should be considered in this child. Some 70% of cases are in girls; 80% of them have the HLA antigen B8 DR3. Clinically a large firm liver is present in over 90% of cases and splenomegaly in 60%. Approximately 25% have other systemic disorders such as vitiligo, arthritis, glomerulonephritis, ulcerative colitis, haemolytic anaemia and iridocyclitis. Serum IgG is always elevated above 16 g/litre; in 15–20% IgM is also elevated. Autoantibodies are present in nearly every case. Overall this boy does not fit well with the above description.

Liver biopsy would be very helpful for diagnosis of both Wilson's disease and ACAH but is contraindicated because of the coagulation defects–these would have to be corrected prior to any procedure. Liver isotope scan might be helpful in demonstrating the size of the liver plus low or normal uptake, indicating an acute necrosis or chronic reparative process respectively.

Acute toxicity from halothane, or other agents, either as a primary or secondary cause is a definite possibility. As a result other anaesthetic agents have come into vogue recently, particularly if multiple anaesthetics are required. Halothane hepatitis is very uncommon in young children. The majority of cases occur in patients who have had more than one exposure to halothane. A specific *in vitro* test for IgG antibodies to halothane-altered liver cell membranes is positive in 70% of cases.

α_1-Antitrypsin deficiency is a rare cause of childhood cirrhosis, but is unlikely here since very few patients develop significant liver disease without a history of obstructive jaundice in infancy.

The easiest way to screen is with a protein electrophoretic strip, where a small α_1 band is seen. The diagnosis is made by protease inhibitor (Pi) phonotyping. The deficiency state phenotypes are PiZ or Pi nul.

Treatment is aimed at correcting the clotting defects and reducing the possibility of hepatic encephalopathy by diet, gut decontamination and H_2 antagonist to prevent bleeding. Hypokalaemia and acid–base imbalance may occur and must be corrected.

Further reading

Inman, W. H. W. and Inman, W. W. (1978). Jaundice after repeated exposure to halothane–reports to the CSM. *British Medical Journal*, **ii**, 1455–6.

Kenna, J. G., Neuberger, J., Mieli-Vergani, G., Mowat, A. P. and Williams, R. (1987). Halothane hepatitis in children. *British Medical Journal*, **294**, 1209–11.

Mowat, A. P. (1987). *Liver Disease in Childhood*, pp. 89–110, 127–34, 151–64, 225–41, 244–55. (London; Butterworths)

Tanner, S. (1989). *Paediatric Hepatology*, pp. 133–60, 165–80, 206–14, 260–1. (Edinburgh; Churchill Livingstone)

Case 51

Answers

1. Enlarged adenoids and tonsils sufficient to cause hypercapnoea with subsequent pulmonary vasoconstriction and hypertension.

Discussion

This child has clinical and cardiographic evidence of right ventricular hypertrophy with pulmonary hypertension and increased right ventricular pressures on catheter studies. There is no evidence of a left-to-right shunt and the right atrial pressure is only minimally raised; this suggests a pulmonary vascular cause of the hypertension. The child was a mouth-breather (suggesting large adenoids), the episodes occurred when the child relaxed, whilst on her back, and upper respiratory tract infections exacerbated the problem. It is possible, therefore, that the airway was sufficiently embarrassed by hypertrophied adenoids and tonsils to cause chronic hypercapnoea and subsequent pulmonary vasoconstriction and hypertension. When the child relaxed the hypertrophied adnexae closed the airway completely. Continued hypertension and increased right-sided pressures result in ventricular hypertrophy; atrial hypertrophy will occur if the ventricular diastolic pressure rises. Vascular response includes an increase in the arterial muscle mass and distal muscular extension. These changes eventually become permanent with irreversible haemodynamic changes. However, diminution of the muscle mass is achieved and haemodynamic equilibrium is restored if the initiating cause is removed promptly, particularly before the age of 2 years.

Pulmonary hypertension also occurs in response to increased pulmonary blood flow as in a left-to-right shunt. Similar physical and haemodynamic consequences occur, again reversible initially. If uncorrected, right-sided pressures may equal and pass systemic pressures, causing reversal of the shunt with cyanosis, the Eisenmenger's syndrome. Careful monitoring of such affected children is, therefore, mandatory.

Further reading

Phelan, P. D., Landau, L. I. and Olinsky, A. (eds) (1990). In *Respiratory Illness in Children*, 3rd edn, pp. 51–2. (Oxford; Blackwell Scientific Publications)

Rabinovitch, M. (1989). Pulmonary hypertension. In *Moss' Heart Disease in Infants, Children and Adolescents*, 4th edn. Ed. by F. H. Adams, G. C. Emmanouilides and T. A. Riemenschneider, pp. 856–72. (Baltimore; Williams & Wilkins)

Case 52

Answers

1. Kugelberg–Welander spinal muscular atrophy.
2. (a) Creatine kinase (CK) activity.
   (b) EMG.
   (c) Muscle biopsy.

Discussion

The main differential diagnosis in this case is between a myopathy and chronic polymyositis. Myopathies frequently present with weakness of the girdle musculature. Early difficulties include lifting, carrying, throwing, combing the hair, running, getting up from a squatting position off the floor or a low chair and climbing stairs. Walking is often unimpaired but patients may have a waddling gait and experience sudden falls due to weakness of the quadriceps. The pattern of muscle wasting is of diagnostic importance; selective atrophy of individual muscles suggests muscular dystrophy while more diffuse wasting and weakness suggest an acquired myopathy or one of the congenital myopathies such as central core disease. The history above is non-specific; discomfort or cramps may occur in myopathic muscles except in metabolic myopathies. This discomfort occurs more commonly if the muscles are hypertrophied such as in Duchenne's muscular dystrophy. Discomfort is more marked on exercise and weakness may well be increased at the end of the day. Limb girdle dystrophy has previously been overdiagnosed and there is now doubt as to whether such a separate entity exists.

Chronic polymyositis which begins insidiously, with increasing weakness over weeks, months or years, is characterized by misery. In contrast myopathic weakness is more diffuse, wasting less pronounced, tendon reflexes preserved and muscle tenderness more common. Other features may be transient rashes, flitting arthralgias and Raynaud's phenomenon. Polymyositis alone, without skin involvement, is relatively uncommon in childhood; however, the skin involvement may be quite subtle. CK is raised in approximately 70% of patients, an EMG will indicate myopathy with fibrillation potentials and muscle biopsy shows fibres undergoing necrosis and phagocytosis with collections of inflammatory cells. Antinuclear antibody (ANA) is often positive. SLE is an outside possibility, but negative ANF and RF results make this unlikely.

Diagnoses that should be considered in a possible myopathy are the benign form of spinal muscular atrophy of Kugelberg–Welander, commonly associated with tremor of the hands; secondly, acid maltase deficiency (type II glycogenosis) which in childhood or adult form, not infantile (Pompe's disease), is very similar. However, the heart and respiratory muscles may be affected leading to respiratory insufficiency. Muscle biopsy is diagnostic, showing fibre atrophy and type grouping in SMA or glycogen storage in acid maltase deficiency.

Uncomfortable or painful muscles at rest occur in other conditions in children. These include trichinosis, which causes muscle pain, weakness and general malaise associated with an eosinophilia; acute myoglobinuric myopathies and myopathies of metabolic bone disease. The former is usually episodic and acute, related to exercise, infection or toxin, while the latter causes only minimal wasting with normal or hyperactive tendon reflexes. CK, EMG and serum calcium may all be normal, but alkaline phosphatase activity is invariably raised.

Further reading

Ansell, B. M. (ed.) (1980). The rarer connective tissue disorders. In *Rheumatic Disorders in Childhood*, pp. 157–212. (London; Butterworths)

Dubowitz, V. (ed.) (1985). *Muscle Biopsy: A Practical Approach*, 2nd edn, pp. 254–86. (London; Baillière Tindall)

Dubowitz, V. (ed.) (1989). *A Colour Atlas of Muscle Disorders in Childhood*, pp. 40–7, 66–86. (London; Wolfe Medical Publications)

Case 53

Answers

1. Digoxin level.
2. Plasma potassium.

Discussion

Digoxin has several effects on the depolarization wave in cardiac muscle. Phase 4, depolarization, has an increased slope, decreasing the time of depolarization and increasing the automaticity of the fibres. This effect of digoxin is a function of intracellular potassium, increased automaticity and excitability of cardiac fibres, eventually causing ectopic beats. In this child the extracellular potassium level was markedly reduced by the diuretic action of theophylline, whereas the digoxin level of 1.5 ng/ml was normal. This combination led to coupled beats. The xanthines, theophylline and 1,3,dimethylxanthine, probably cause a diuresis by inhibiting the reabsorption of sodium and chloride in the proximal convoluted tubule. This allows greater sodium–potassium exchange in the distal convoluted tubule.

The cellular basis of action of the xanthines has not been fully elucidated. Three possible actions have been suggested. The first relates to the translocation of intracellular calcium. This may account for the stimulation of cardiac and striated muscle. However, smooth muscle, especially bronchial muscle, is relaxed. Secondly, the xanthines inhibit phosphodiesterase, increasing intracellular cyclic adenosine monophosphate (AMP); this may account for excitation of the central nervous system producing decreased tiredness and more efficient functioning. The third mechanism is the block of adenosine receptors. Adenosine may act via cyclic AMP or be totally independent of it.

Other less well-established hypotheses of action include potentiation of inhibitors of prostaglandin synthesis and the reduction of uptake/metabolism of catecholamines in non-neuronal tissues. The effects of adenosine include dilatation of the blood vessels, especially coronary and cerebral, and slowing of the rate of discharge of the cardiac pacemaker cells and some neurons in the central nervous system. However, the clinical effects of theophylline include constriction of the cerebral vasculature and stimulation of cardiac fibres and the central nervous system. There must obviously be complex cellular interactions before the clinical effects of theophylline are manifest.

Further reading

Isles, A. F. and Newth, C. J. L. (1985). Respiratory pharmacology. In *Textbook of Pediatric Clinical Pharmacology*, Ed. by S. M. McLeod and I. C. Radde, pp. 197–9. (Littleton; PSG Publications)

Olley, P. and Rabinovitch, M. (1985). Drugs affecting the cardiovascular system. In *Textbook of Pediatric Clinical Pharmacology*, Ed. by S. M. McLeod and I. C. Radde, pp. 148–58. (Littleton; PSG Publications)

Case 54

Answers

1. (a) CT scan.
   (b) Jejunal biopsy.

    (c) Skull X-ray.
    (d) Serum triiodothyronine and thyroxine.
2. (a) Hypothalamic tumour (diencephalic syndrome of child-
       hood).
    (b) Psychosocial deprivation.
3. (a) Shunt procedure for hydrocephalus.
    (b) Radiotherapy.

Discussion

Here is a case of marked failure to thrive in a happy, alert, almost euphoric child. Even when the calorie intake is sufficient, weight gain is poor. Various diagnoses have been excluded, i.e. cystic fibrosis, congenital heart disease, chronic infection, particularly pulmonary or renal, by putting together the examination and investigations. Malabsorption is unlikely, the haemaglobin level and 1-hour xylose are normal, but there is a low albumin and enteropathogenic *Escherichia coli* in the stool with no history of diarrhoea. In this situation a jejunal biopsy is indicated to rule out an enteropathy.

The differential diagnosis lies between psychosocial deprivation and an intracranial lesion. There are certainly sufficient factors in the family and social history to fit with emotional deprivation, but this child always appeared very happy and on admission to hospital did not gain weight as expected with a change of environment and regular feeding. His height on the 25th centile and weight on the 3rd are also against this diagnosis. One would expect short stature in keeping with the weight.

An intracranial lesion is therefore the most likely diagnosis. In view of the history and absence of neurological signs apart from nystagmus, a hypothalamic tumour or one in the floor of the third ventricle is most likely. When the tumour is in the anterior wall of the third ventricle the infants are either anorexic or have a voracious appetite and become progressively emaciated while remaining bright, happy and active. Hydrocephalus may be symptomless, skin depigmentation is usual, hypotension and hypoglycaemia may occur; growth hormone levels have been reported as grossly elevated. With tumours of other areas of the hypothalmus the optic nerves and chiasma are encroached on early. This results in visual field defects and optic atrophy. In this case the nystagmus may have been due to disturbed macular vision secondary to the tumour but optic atrophy was not noted.

Hydrocephalus is progressive as a result of third ventricle invasion and requires treatment. The tumour is an astrocytoma and since it is inaccessible to surgery, treatment is with radiotherapy.

Useful investigations are limited. Skull X-rays may show separation of the sutures; visual fields would be extremely difficult, if not impossble in such a child; but a CT or MRI scan is mandatory.

Hyperthyroidism is a possibility, but in this age group very rare, especially with no goitre or eye signs. It is most common in adolescent females who develop thyroid antibodies. Serum levels of triiodothyronine and thyroxine are usually elevated.

Further reading

Bain, H. W., Darte, J. H. M., Keith, W. S. and Krayff, E. (1966). The diencephalic syndrome of early infancy due to silent brain tumours with special reference to treatment. *Paediatrics*, **38**, 473.

Brett, E. M. (1991). *Paediatric Neurology*, pp. 525–6. (Edinburgh; Churchill Livingstone)

Case 55

Answers

1. (a) Typhoid.
   (b) Paratyphoid.
2. (a) Blood culture.
   (b) Widal's agglutination test.
   (c) Stool culture.
   (d) Urine culture.
3. (a) Chloramphenicol or ciprofloxacin.
   (b) Co-trimoxazole.
   (c) Amoxycillin.

Discussion

Typhoid in children can present in a number of unusual ways, often just as a pyrexia of unknown origin (PUO) with no accompanying diarrhoea. This child presents a fairly typical picture of early typhoid with abdominal pain, fever, headache and cough. The signs on examination are generally non-specific. Meningism is sometimes present, together with mental confusion, but examination of the CSF is usually normal. It is well-recognized that there can be positive findings on clinical examination of the chest, but the chest X-ray is often surprisingly clear. Leukopenia is common in typhoid, although it is also present in a viral infection or overwhelming bacterial infection.

Jaundice can be one of the initial presentations of typhoid fever due to haemolysis and anaemia is common. Raised transaminase activities are often non-specific findings.

As the illness proceeds, the temperature rises often in typical 'staircase' fashion. Towards the end of the first week, the patient becomes more toxic, sometimes confused with increasing abdominal pain, distension and tenderness; the diarrhoea starts and rose spots may appear mainly on the trunk. Although convulsions are not very common they do occur, especially in children. More common complications are gastrointestinal haemorrhage and perforation.

Paratyphoid fever can present with a similar picture to typhoid fever but is usually less severe. Lassa fever, only found in Nigeria, also presents with a similar course.

Other diagnoses that may be considered are *Shigella* dysentery which generally presents with diarrhoea and possibly dehydration, but a young child may be toxic and have meningism. Blood in the stool with abdominal pain also occurs with giardiasis, *Campylobacter* and amoebiasis, but the children are not markedly pyrexial and meningism does not occur. *Yersinia* enterocolitis gives a clinical picture varying from mesenteric adenitis to acute diarrhoea of brief duration. Recently *Cryptosporidium* has been recognized as an intestinal pathogen causing diarrhoea, abdominal pain and flatulence lasting about 10 days on average but without the severe constitutional symptoms described in this child.

Salmonella typhi should be grown from a blood culture. It can also be isolated from the stools and urine but this does not prove the diagnosis unequivocally since the patient may be a carrier with an unrelated illness, although this coincidence is unusual. A rising titre on Widal's agglutination test in a patient who has not received typhoid vaccine recently is good evidence in favour of typhoid fever.

Chloramphenicol has been the mainstay of treatment but there is increasing incidence of chloramphenicol resistance. Ciprofloxacin is now the drug of choice in adults. There have been reports of joint problems in children but ciprofloxacin will probably, out of necessity, become the drug of choice in all age groups. Co-trimoxazole has been used fairly extensively for fully sensitive organisms, amoxycillin is also effective and has been used in the treatment of the chronic carrier state.

Further reading

Manson-Bann, P. E. C. and Bell, D. R. (1987). *Typhoid Fever in Manson's Tropical Diseases*, pp. 194–206. (London; Baillière Tindall)

Marks, M. I. (1985). *Paediatric Infectious Diseases for the Practitioner*, pp. 155–6; 725–7. (New York; Springer-Verlag)

Case 56

Answers

1. Poliomyelitis.
2. (a) Stool and pharyngeal washings for viruses.
   (b) CSF for microscopy, protein, viral and bacterial cultures.
   (c) Paired serum antibody titres for polioviruses.
   (d) Motor nerve conduction studies.
3. (a) Bed rest for child during acute phase.
   (b) Report case to District Medical Officer.
   (c) Make sure that encampment is fully immunized (this should be done by Community Health Department).
   (d) Watch for respiratory and bulbar complications.
   (e) Physiotherapy in recovery phase.

Discussion

Other diagnoses which should be considered here besides poliomyelitis are Guillain–Barré syndrome (GBS), peripheral neuropathy and acute viral infections including aseptic meningitis. In GBS there is often a preceding viral illness but the paralysis usually progresses slowly over 1–2 weeks, while in polio paralysis progresses quickly; the final extent can usually be assessed in 48–72 hours. Secondly, in GBS there is symmetrical paralysis, usually sensory symptoms, a high CSF protein up to 7 g/litre and low cell count, while in polio paralysis is classically asymmetrical and there are no sensory symptoms. CSF protein is normal and cell count consistent with viral meningitis. Both conditions have muscle pain preceding paralysis; this can vary considerably in its severity but is usually more marked in GBS. When paralysis is more symmetrical than in this case, transverse myelitis has to be considered; in this case a clear motor and sensory level is often found.

Peripheral neuropathy of acute onset may also be due to porphyria (which is most unlikely in a child so young), diphtheria (in which aseptic meningitis does not develop and which generally causes severe constitutional upset), toxins such as lead and other heavy metals, drugs such as isoniazid or vincristine and serum sickness after immunization.

Signs of aseptic meningitis together with weakness and flaccidity, sometimes associated with spasm and tenderness, occur rarely in some Coxsackie B and echovirus infections. If there is somnolence, disorientation and coma plus an absence of fever or neck stiffness at the time of onset of paralysis and complete recovery of weakness in 7–10 days, the diagnosis of poliovirus infection is very doubtful. Adenoviruses are infrequent causes of meningitis or encephalitis; mumps virus is the most frequently identified cause of aseptic meningitis; there is no associated paralysis.

Diagnosis is by isolation of the virus. Stools are the best material. The best way is to inoculate faecal material into monkey kidney to grow the virus; throat washings are of use in the first week. It is rarely isolated from the CSF·and a lumbar punture may increase paralysis once the paralytic stage has been reached. Paralysis is more common at sites of recent trauma; for example, bulbar palsy is more likely after tonsillectomy. There is a fourfold rise in antibody titre to the isolated virus in acute and convalescent serum. Lastly, motor nerve conduction velocity is slowed in GBS, which distinguishes it from polio.

In a sporadic case such as this, reporting of the case to Public Health Department is of primary importance. This could be either a wild virus or an attenuated virus from another child who has recently been immunized. It is important that the gypsy camp population is screened and immunized, since this will stop the spread of the virus. For the child, nursing care in the acute phase consists of keeping the full range of movement in the limbs, prevention of bed sores and chest infection, watching for respiratory and bulbar paralysis. Once the acute phase of increasing paralysis has passed, active physiotherapy to try to regain as much movement as possible should be given.

Further reading

Brett, E. M. (1991). *Paediatric Neurology*, pp. 617–18. (Edinburgh; Churchill Livingstone)

Marks, M. I. (1985). *Pediatric Infectious Diseases for the Practitioner*, pp. 611–15; 621–6. (New York; Springer-Verlag)

Ramsay, A. M. and Emond, R. T. D. (1957). Poliomyelitis. In *Infectious Diseases*, pp. 120–32. (London; Heinemann)

Case 57

Answers

1. Hyponatraemia.
2. (a) Serum sodium level.
   (b) Serum osmolality

Discussion

The mother had received a large volume of hypotonic fluid for her size and, in addition, had had an oxytocin infusion. Oxytocin has a modest intrinsic antidiuretic action, causing expansion of the maternal and, therefore, the fetal extracellular fluid compartments. The term newborn infant has a low renal blood flow and glomerular filtration rate, even when corrected for surface area. This reduces the ability of the kidney to excrete a water load. The child was born at approximately 36 weeks' gestation. However, his birth weight was 3rd centile for 36 weeks but at the 50th centile for 32 weeks' gestation. This prematurity would effect a concomitant reduction in renal maturity. The serum sodium in this child was 116 mmol/litre. Serum osmolality would be low but would not indicate which of the osmotically active agents was so deficient. The treatment is to correct the serum sodium concentration with hypertonic sodium infusion over 6–10 hours.

Maturation of the kidney is both anatomical and hormonal. Renal blood flow and glomerular filtration rate increase rapidly.

220

The neonatal loop of Henle is shorter than the adult, permitting a maximal urinary concentration of 50–60% of the adult, despite the slow fluid flow facilitating solute reabsorption. Growth of the loop of Henle is rapid in the first 9 months of life.

The distal convuluted tubule and collecting ducts are relatively insensible to ADH. ADH acts via cyclic AMP, which rises only modestly in the neonate. Again maturation occurs rapidly in the first few months of life. The immature kidney, therefore, is inefficient at excreting either a high solute load or high water load.

Further reading

Aperia, A. (1987). The adaptive capacity of the newborn. In *Pediatric Nephrology*. 2nd edn, Ed. by M. A. Holliday, T. M. Barrett and R. L. Vernier, pp. 12–7. (Baltimore; Williams & Wilkins)
de Wardener, H. E. (ed). (1985). *The Kidney*, 5th edn, pp. 56–83; 314–18. (London; Churchill Livingstone)

Case 58

Answers

1. Immunoglobulins.
2. (a) Appropriate antimicrobial treatment following infection screen, taking into account any known cultures and sensitivities.
   (b) Correct fluid and electrolytes balance, then consider nutrition with either an elemental diet or parenteral feeding.
   (c) Irradiated blood transfusion.
   (d) Gammaglobulin.
   (e) Bone marrow transplant.
3. Severe combined immune deficiency (SCID).

Discussion

The relevant points in this patient's history are the recurrent infections and failure to thrive, with gastrointestinal symptoms in the presence of lymphopenia. Any child with this combination of symptoms should be investigated immunologically. Those presenting in the first 6 months of life are likely to have a defect of cell-mediated immunity at least. This is supported by the absolute lymphopenia, which can be further broken down into B and T cell numbers, but more importantly, function. In this child T cell function was inadvertently tested by trying to do chromosome analysis. The lymphocytes would not respond to PHA, one of the commonly used mitogens; this can be tested further by delayed type hypersensitivity reaction to either intradermal PHA or *Candida* antigen. Immunoglobulin levels G, A and M were all very low. These can be difficult to interpret in the first year because of the passive transfer of material IgG before birth, decreasing slowly over the first 3 months. Congenital forms of antibody deficiency usually present with recurrent infections, particularly of the respiratory tract, between 4 months and 2 years.

SCID (deficiency of B and T lymphocytes) can be autosomal recessive, sex-linked or occasionally sporadic with a male to female ratio of 4 : 1. It usually presents during the first few months of life with infections resulting in diarrhoea, failure to thrive, pneumonia, skin sepsis, oral and systemic candidiasis. Infecting organisms are both common and opportunisitic, for example, *Pneumocystis carinii*, RSV, CMV, adenovirus, *Giardia lamblia*, *Cryptosporidium* and rotavirus. All these infections are particularly resistant to treatment; the diarrhoea and failure to thrive are unresponsive to elimination of disaccharidases, dairy products and other foods. Sometimes a graft-versus-host reaction in the form of an erythematous rash is seen either from maternal lymphocytes or following an unirradiated blood transfusion. Clinically there is no lymphoid tissue including thymus, no hepatosplenomegaly, an absolute lymphopenia and low or absent immunoglobulins.

In contrast to infants with SCID, boys with X-linked hypogammaglobulinaemia have lymph nodes, tonsils and adenoids, a thymus on chest X-ray, and no lymphopenia. B and T lymphocyte markers will show lack of surface immunoglobulins on B cells but normal numbers of T cells; T cell function is intact. Other X-linked conditions are chronic granulomatous disease which generally presents with recurrent skin infections, osteomyelitis and hepatosplenomegaly; Wiskott–Aldrich syndrome presenting with infections, thrombocytopenia and eczema.

The acquired immune deficiency syndrome (AIDS) is now probably the most important immune deficiency disorder and must be borne in mind even in such a young child where the infection could be congenital. Measurement of HIV antibodies should be done after appropriate consultation with the parents.

Treatment of an immune-compromised patient follows general lines at first with eradication of infection as far as possible. Initially broad-spectrum antibiotics, an aminoglycoside and an antipseudomonal penicillin may be used. Antibiotics are changed to take into account any positive cultures and sensitivities. Routine prophylaxis for *Candida* is given, usually with oral amphotericin and for pneumocystis with co-trimoxazole.

Secondly, it is important to regain fluid and electrolyte balance followed by improved nutrition prior to carrying out a possible curative procedure such as bone marrow transplantation. Parenteral feeding would probably be necessary at first but indwelling intravenous catheters give an increased incidence of systemic infection, particularly candidiasis. Hence enteral nutrition with an elemental or elimination diet should be started at the earliest opportunity to cater for any intolerances.

All blood products must be irradiated, otherwise fatal graft-versus-host reactions may occur. Gammaglobulin may be useful. Bone marrow transplant from a histocompatible sibling is the only 'cure' for this condition and is worth undertaking even in unfavourable circumstances if the child is very unwell, since it may be its only chance for life.

Further Reading

Haeney, M. (1991). The detection and management of primary immunodeficiency. In *Recent Advances in Paediatrics* no. 9 Ed. by T. J. David, pp. 21–39. (Edinburgh; Churchill Livingstone)

Walker-Smith, J. (1988). *Diseases of the Small Intestine in Childhood*, 3rd Edn., pp. 127–33. (London; Butterworths)

Watson, J. G. and Bird, A. G. (1990). *Handbook of Immunological Investigations in Children*, pp. 7–44. (Bristol; Wright)

Case 59

Answers

1. Postnatal extrahepatic biliary atresia.
2. α_1-antitrypsin deficiency.

Discussion

This infant has evidence of a worsening cholestatic jaundice first noticed shortly after birth. Conjugated hyperbilirubinaemia has multiple causes including infection, inborn errors of metabolism and biliary atresia. No evidence of pre- or postnatal infection was detected; this, however, does not preclude a diagnosis of hepatitis as many cases have no cause determined. No evidence of galactosaemia or fructosaemia was found. Again this does not preclude these diagnoses as patients may not have galactosuria or fructosuria for several months. Obviously the patient must have ingested the relevant disaccharide.

Liver biopsy revealed proliferation of the bile ductules with an inflammatory exudate. This histology is compatible with extrahepatic biliary atresia and α_1-antitrypsin deficiency. Multinucleated giant cells are more commonly associated with hepatitis, but may be seen in both conditions. The infant was of normal birth weight, whereas the majority of patients with α_1-antitrypsin deficiency are of low birth weight.

Congenital biliary atresia produces a similar histological appearance, but is unlikely as this child was not jaundiced from birth. Postnatal biliary atresia is, therefore, more likely.

The incidence of extrahepatic biliary atresia is approximately 1 in 14 000 live births; the aetiology is unknown. It is postulated that the precipitating insult initiates a sclerosing inflammatory lesion in the ductular tissues. This may occur in fetal, perinatal or early postnatal life, allowing, as in this case, a picture of hepatitis superseded by that of atresia. Some 25% of cases of extrahepatic biliary atresia have associated congenital malformations; however, no one system is particularly implicated. Diagnosis should be made rapidly as results indicate that operative procedures should be performed before 80 days of age to carry a reasonable prognosis. Diagnosis should be made on a combination of clinical suspicion, a Technetium 99m DISIDA scan demonstrating abnormal radiolabel excretion and a characteristic biopsy. Ultrasound is helpful in determining the presence of large extrahepatic masses but will not detect conclusively the absence of a biliary tree. Laparotomy may be necessary to determine a definitive diagnosis.

The operation of choice is hepatic portoenterostomy, allowing bile to drain into a blind-ending loop of jejunum. There is no effective medical treatment and death usually supervenes within 2 years without surgery. There is a significant incidence of ascending cholangitis after this procedure.

α_1-Antitrypsin deficiency is a rare disease causing hepatitis with subsequent cirrhosis and emphysema. α_1-Antitrypsin is an acute-phase protein; levels rise during infection, surgery or pregnancy. There are several phenotypes. PiMM is the most common normal combination. Those suffering from the disease commonly have either the phenotype PiZZ or Pinull, with no α_1-antitrypsin. Not all patients with deficiency suffer symptoms, and other genetic control factors have been postulated to explain these observations.

Initially the liver biopsy may resemble that of extrahepatic biliary atresia. However, after 12 weeks of age characteristic intracellular deposits are noted. Clinical presentation is varied, ranging from mild icterus with slow weight gain to marked failure to thrive, vomiting, hypotension and septicaemia. Survivors of the acute phase later develop cirrhosis. The onset of pulmonary symptoms usually occurs in the third or fourth decade; however, a few cases of childhood and adolescent onset have been reported. Liver transplantation may offer some hope.

Further reading

Phelan, P. D., Landau, L. I., Olinsky, A. (eds). (1990). *Respiratory Illness in Children*, 3rd edn. pp. 93–4. (Oxford; Blackwell Scientific Publications)

Tanner, S. (ed.) (1989). *Paediatric Hepatology*, pp. 50–63; 88–95. (London; Churchill Livingstone)

Wigglesworth, J. S. (ed.) (1984). *Perinatal Pathology*, pp. 311–6. (Philadelphia; W. B. Saunders)

Case 60

Answers

1. G6PD deficiency.
2. (a) G6PD level in RBCs.
   (b) Fluorescent spot test.
   (c) Hb electrophoresis.
   (d) Family studies, especially G6PD in mother.
   (e) Coombs test.
   (f) Chest X-ray.
   (g) Liver function tests.

3. (a) Sulphonamides.
   (b) Nitrofurantoin.
   (c) Fava beans.
   (d) Primaquine.
   (e) Naphthalene.

Discussion

This boy presents a picture of acute haemolysis with anaemia, reticulocytosis and jaundice. There are also features of intravascular haemolysis with fragmented RBCs and haemoglobulinuria (dark urine); urobilinogen is not dark. Heinz bodies demonstrate oxidant haemolysis, being aggregates of oxidized and denatured Hb attached to the red cell membrane. The absence of spherocytes suggests that the haemolysis is not autoimmune, these being the characteristic morphological features in warm antibody haemolytic anaemia. Any other diagnosis that might be considered, such as hepatitis, nephritis, parvovirus infection with marrow aplasia, or leukaemia, does not fit the clinical picture, i.e. normal coloured stools, normal urea and electrolytes, low blood pressure and good marrow response to anaemia.

The most common cause of oxidant haemolysis is G6PD deficiency, especially in a boy of near-oriental or Mediterranean origin. It is inherited as a sex-linked recessive. Heamolysis may occur spontaneously but generally is secondary to drugs such as primaquine and sulphonamides. Fava beans, a staple dietary component of Mediterranean people, cause haemolysis, the condition being called favism. This boy had been seen eating a small piece of mothball (naphthalene), also well-recognized to cause haemolysis. Infections such as hepatitis or pneumonia may cause haemolytic episodes in deficient individuals, hence the relevance of a chest X-ray and liver function tests.

Diagnosis is best made by measuring the level of G6PD in the red cells. However, a good screening test is a fluorescent spot test which is based on the reduction by haemolysate of nicotinamide adenine dinucleotide (NADP) to NADPH which fluoresces under ultraviolet light. G6PD-deficient red cells cannot produce the reduced NADPH and thus no fluorescent spot appears on the filter paper. Other investigations which are appropriate for any patient with haemolytic anaemia are the Coombs test which, if positive, means autoantibodies are present; Hb electrophoresis to look for unstable haemoglobin, e.g. Koln Hb; family studies, especially for G6PD in mother, but also for any other possible cause of haemolysis.

Other causes of intravascular haemolysis are paroxysmal nocturnal haemoglobinuria (PNH) and paroxysmal cold haemoglobinuria, both very unusual in this age group, and mechanical haemolysis from a prosthetic heart valve. The history does not suggest any of these diagnoses.

Further Reading

Nathan, D. G. and Oski, F. A. (1987). *Haematology of Infancy and Childhood*, 3rd Edn, pp. 583–612. (Philadelphia; Saunders)

Sullivan, D. W. and Glader, B. E. (1980). Erythrocyte enzyme disorders in children. *Pediatric Clinics of North America*, **27**, 449–52.

Case 61

Answers

1. (a) Tracheo-oesophageal fistula.
   (b) Oesophageal stricture, e. g. vascular ring.
   (c) Achalasia of the cardia.
   (d) Abnormal oesophageal motility.
   (e) Hiatus hernia.
   (f) Tracheo-oesophageal cleft.
   (g) Pharyngeal pouch.
2. (a) Videoradiography during barium swallow.
   (b) Bronchoscopy.
   (c) Oesophageal motility studies.

Discussion

Recurrent chest infections have a multiplicity of aetiologies. Such possibilities include a left-to-right shunt, lung parenchymal damage, immune deficiency and recurrent inhalation. Many aspects of this history suggest inhalation. Coughing occurred intermittently from birth, sometimes associated with feeding. Eventually the cough became persistent and wheezing was noted. Chest X-ray changes were restricted to both lower lobes, which are the areas affected by inhalation while upright. Corroborative evidence included normal immunoglobulins, sweat test, stool trypsin activity and absence of a cardiovascular abnormality.

A common cause of inhalation is palatal and pharyngeal incoordination, especially in the premature baby or in those with neurological damage. At 37 weeks' gestation, poor palatal control may occur. However, co-ordination should rapidly develop in the absence of neurological deficit, as in this child who is developmentally and neurologically normal. Inhalation may occur secondary to congenital abnormalities. Tracheo-oesophageal fistula permits the passage of foodstuffs to the lungs. A large fistula would cause catastrophic results which may be fatal; if the lumen is narrow only small amounts of fluid pass. As this continues the reflex coughing may diminish and it may be difficult to relate the episodes to feeding. A rare variation of abnormal foregut development is a tracheo-oesophageal cleft, where the two structures fail to separate. The cleft may be insignificant or extend to the pharynx or bronchi.

Stasis or interruption of the passage of food, as in achalasia, stricture of the oesophagus or abnormal oesophageal motility, facilitates inhalation. Regurgitation into the oropharynx permitted by a hiatus hernia, especially when recumbent, allows inhalation. Rarely a pharyngeal pouch may be implicated.

The association of coughing with feeding suggests the most likely diagnoses are a tracheo-oesophageal fistula, achalasia or stricture of the oesophagus.

Diagnosis of the 'H' tracheo-oesophageal fistula, which accounts for only 4% of such abnormalities, may present severe problems. Videoradiography during a swallow may or may not outline the fistula transiently. Bronchoscopy, however, should reveal the abnormal opening. Rarely, fistulas may occur from the oesophagus or stomach to the bronchi.

The most common form of tracheo-oesophageal fistula is with a blind-ending proximal oesophageal pouch and a fistula from the trachea to the distal oesophagus. Diagnosis should be made rapidly as the infant can swallow nothing. Surgery is indicated in all these abnormalities. Unfortunately, even though anastomosis may be possible, oesophageal peristalsis is usually abnormal, with resulting repeated inhalation. Approximately 20% of cases are associated with other congenital abnormalities, usually in the renal, cardiovascular or gastrointestinal systems.

228

Further reading

Cudmore, R. E. (1990). Oesophageal atresia and tracheo-oesophageal fistula. In *Neonatal Surgery*, 3rd edn, Ed. by J. Lister and I. M. Irving, pp. 231–48. (London; Butterworths)

Phelan, P. D., Landau, L. I. and Olinsky, A. (eds) (1990). *Respiratory Illness in Children*, 3rd edn, pp. 234–43. (Oxford; Blackwell Scientific Publications)

Spitz, L. (1988). Surgical emergencies in the first few weeks of life. In *Harries' Paediatric Gastroenterology*, 2nd edn, Ed. by P. J. Milla and D. P. R. Muller, pp. 83–6. (London; Churchill Livingstone)

Case 62

Answers

1. (a) Reducing substances.
   (b) Red cell enzymes.
   (c) Insulin levels, ketone bodies and intermediate metabolites of gluconeogenesis taken at a time of proven hypoglycaemia.
   (d) Urinary amino acids.
   (e) Toxoplasmosis, others, rubella, CMV, herpes (TORCH) antibodies.
2. Von Gierke's disease (type I glycogenosis).

Discussion

Neonatal hypoglycaemia, usually defined as a blood glucose level of less than 1.6 mmol/litre in the term infant, is a common problem. Several categories of infants are 'at risk', including the preterm, small for gestational age and infants of diabetic mothers. Certain perinatal catastrophes such as IVH, rhesus incompatability and neonatal cold injury also predispose to hypoglycaemia. Hypoglycaemia is also reported in the presence of polycythaemia, but it is apparent rather than real. This infant is an apparently healthy full-term child who rapidly develops resistant hypoglycaemia, shortly after being fed. Although early, it is important to exclude galactosaemia.

The older sibling died in the early neonatal period, suggesting an inherited disorder, possibly of amino acid metabolism or metabolite storage. A mild metabolic acidosis was noted and also hepatosplenomegaly; these features would be explained by a glycogen storage disease, especially type I–von Gierke's disease.

The determination of insulin levels during hypoglycaemia would be useful to differentiate failure of production from causes with excess insulin, such as nesidioblastosis, B cell adenomatosis and erythroblastosis fetalis. Ketone bodies, lactic acid and intermediate metabolites are absent in the presence of raised insulin levels. Somatostatin has been used to control the hypoglycaemia of nesidioblastosis in the short to middle term rather than proceed to subtotal pancreatectomy immediately. Organomegaly is not associated with these pancreatic abnormalities.

Von Gierke's disease is caused by a deficiency of glucose-6-phosphatase which inhibits the release of glucose from glycogen or gluconeogenesis. The symptoms, therefore, relate to the subsequent hypoglycaemia. The infantile presentation is the least common but most severe variant. Control of the hypoglycaemia may be extremely difficult, occasionally requiring intravenous alimentation or a portocaval shunt. Even so, the mortality rate in the first year of life is high. Presentation may be via apnoeic episodes, vomiting or failure to thrive; convulsions may occur. Fatty infiltration of the liver is progressive and a bleeding diathesis with thrombocytosis may be a complicating factor.

Biochemical changes secondary to the hypoglycaemia include hyperlipidaemia from lipolysis, ketosis and lactic acidosis and hyperuricaemia, probably due to a renal transport defect secondary to hyperlactataemia.

Increasing glycogen deposition causes progressive hepatosplenomegaly and bony changes with thinning of the cortex and widening of the medulla.

The combination of the above biochemical abnormalities suggests the diagnosis, which is verified by liver biopsy.

Treatment is with small frequent meals with a high carbohydrate content.

Bone marrow transplantation is being used for inborn errors of metabolism, with variable results.

Further reading

Aynsley-Green, A. (1988). The management of islet cell dysregulation syndromes in infancy and childhood. *Zeitschrift für Kinderchirugie*, **43**, 267–72.

Levy, H. L. (1984). Inborn errors of carbohydrate metabolism. In *Schaffer's Diseases of the Newborn*, 5th edn, Ed. by M. E. Avery and H. W. Taeusch, pp. 534–5. (Philadelphia; W. B. Saunders)

Stacey, T. E, Macnab, A. and Strang, L. B. (1980). Recent work on the treatment of type 1 glycogen storage disease. In *Inherited Disorders of Carbohydrate Metabolism*, Ed. by D. Burman, J. B. Holton and C. A. Pennod, pp. 315–24. (London; MTP Publications)

Case 63

Answers

1. X-linked nephrogenic diabetes insipidus (DI).
2. (a) Urine osmolality.
   (b) Response to vasopressin or desmopressin on urine osmolality.
   (c) Further family history of male children, especially infant, deaths.
   (d) Further history of polyuria and thirst in the patient and any other family member.
   (e) Plasma ADH when patient is hyperosmolar.
3. (a) Low protein and sodium, high carbohydrate and fat diet.
   (b) Adequate water intake.
   (c) Chlorothiazide with potassium supplements.
   (d) Indomethacin.

Discussion

This little boy is dehydrated, hypernatraemic, normokalaemic and markedly hyperosmolar, although apparently still passing urine. Gastroenteritis in an infant may result in hypernatraemic dehydration but this is generally associated with injudicious feeds. This child is said to have been on clear fluids. The content is not mentioned, but this suggests that medical help has already been sought. The history of failure to thrive and repeated pyrexial episodes of unexplained aetiology suggests a metabolic or immune abnormality. Immune defects are rather unlikey since no specific infection has been found. In a child of 7 months who is already failing to thrive, this would be very unusual.

Hypernatraemia and dehydration may be caused by excessive salt intake when dehydrated, as mentioned above, too much water loss, or too much salt retention, which is difficult to explain in the face of dehydration. The differential diagnosis is between DI, both hypothalamic and nephrogenic in origin, primary or pseudohyperaldosteronism (Liddle's syndrome). The latter two are both very rare and may produce severe growth retardation plus polydipsia, polyuria, intermittent paralysis, fatigue or muscular weakness, some of these symtoms resulting from potassium depletion. Serum sodium, pH and bicarbonate concentrations are all raised; potassium and chloride levels are low. Hypertension always occurs secondary to the raised intravascular volume from sodium and water retention, and there may be cardiomegaly plus retinopathy. In primary aldosteronism, the aldosterone level is high and renin low while in pseudoaldosteronism, both levels are low.

No history is given of polyhydramnios in pregnancy, polydipsia or polyuria, but would probably be forthcoming if asked for. DI, both hypothalamic and nephrogenic in origin, may present in infancy with polyuria, polydipsia and dehydration. The initial clue to nephrogenic DI often is repeated episodes of unexplained fever. A family history of similar problems in males, since it is usually X-linked, would support the diagnosis. In both types of DI severe dehydration may present in infancy with constipation, vomiting and fever, resulting in marked failure to thrive because of inadequate calorie intake secondary to the severe thirst for water. In hypothalamic DI, hyperthermia, rapid weight loss and collapse are common in infancy. In both types severe dehydration may result in brain damage. In nephrogenic DI the severity of retardation is related to the age at which the diagnosis is made and therapy started. This is due not only to dehydration but also to hypernatraemia. Hypernatraemia appears to be a fairly constant feature since maximum urine osmolality is usually 80–150 mosmol/litre. Any solute load such as sodium, chloride and urea thus requires a large urine volume in which to be excreted. In hypothalamic DI urine osmolality is usually between 50 and 200 mosmol/litre, but during periods of severe dehydration may rise to 300 mosmol/litre. Serum osmolality is normal with adequate hydration; hypernatraemia is not a constant feature as in nephrogenic DI. Nephrogenic DI should be suspected when there is persistently hypotonic urine in the face of clinical dehydration, or an elevated serum sodium or osmolality. The critical test is the lack of rise in urine osmolality in response to vasopressin (or the synthetic DDVAP) in this situation. Increased urine osmolality would occur in hypothalamic DI. It is possible to measure plasma ADH by radioimmunoassay prior to giving DDAVP.

In nephrogenic DI, the distal tubules and collecting ducts are insensitive to ADH, thus diffusion of luminal water into the hypertonic medullary interstitium is markedly reduced. The exact reason for this is unknown and may involve various breaks in the pathway by which ADH increases the tubular permeability to water. This involves adenosine triphosphate dephosphorylation to cyclic AMP catalysed by adenyl cyclase and ADH. There are many other factors that influence this chain of events. These include renal prostaglandins, hypercalcaemia and hypokalaemia. The latter two are both causes of polyuria. Primary polydipsia (habitual water drinking) can produce hypokalaemia and partial lack of tubular permeability to water. A prolonged water deprivation test may be required to show increasing urine osmolality. Other causes of polyuria are a result of the primary defect being in the medullary solute gradient. Examples are: chronic renal failure, chronic obstructive nephropathy, medullary cystic disease, Fanconi's syndrome and interstitial nephropathy.

Treatment is aimed at (1) giving sufficient fluids and calories; (2) reducing the solute load; and (3) trying to reduce the urine volume. A diet high in carbohydrate and fat, but low in protein and salt (which increase the solute load) should be given, always with a high water intake. Diuretics, such as chlorothiazide in combination with a low sodium intake, appear to reduce the urine volume by up to 50%. The mechanism is not fully understood but it appears that together they produce a state of sodium depletion, which leads to a greater reabsorption of salt and water than normal in the proximal tubule. This alone appears to reduce the volume of fluid delivered to the loop of Henle and distal tubule. Potassium supplements will obviously be necessary. Indomethacin, as a prostaglandin inhibitor, is useful and can be used in combination with a thiazide diuretic.

Hirschsprung's disease has been suggested as one of the differential diagnoses here. This could be true with the history of constipation and intermittent diarrhoea. Vomiting may occur secondary to partial intestinal obstruction. Severe dehydration would be most unlikely unless fulminant enterocolitis was present, in which case electrolyte losses should have occurred and hypertraemia would not occur. A 7-month-old child who is failing to thrive due to Hirschsprung's disease would have moderate-to-severe disease and marked abdominal distension. In view of the symptoms, signs and investigations, a diagnosis of Hirschsprung's disease cannot be justified.

Further reading

Perheentupa, J. (1981). The neurohypophysis and water regulation. In *Clinical Paediatric Endocrinology* Ed. by C. G. D. Brook, p. 315. (Oxford; Blackwell Scientific Publications)

Postlethwaite, R. J. (1986). *Clinical Paediatric Nephrology*, pp. 12–13; 98–101; 248–50; 425. (Bristol; Wright)

Stern, P. (1979). Nephrogenic defects of urinary concentration. In *Diseases of the Kidney*, Vol. II, Ed. by C. M. Edelmann, pp. 978–93. (Philadelphia; Little, Brown)

Case 64

Answers

1. Pericarditis, acute.
2. (a) Bacterial secondary to chest infection or septicaemia, e.g. staphylococal, streptococcal, pneumococcal.
   (b) Viral, e.g. coxsackie B.
   (c) Tuberculosis.
   (d) Rheumatoid disease.
   (e) Malignant infiltration of the heart.
3. (a) ECG.
   (b) Chest X-ray and screening.
   (c) Ultrasound echocardiogram.
   (d) Blood culture.
   (e) Pericardial tap–fluid for microscopy, bacterial and viral cultures.
   (f) Viral studies.
   (g) Mantoux test.
   (h) Countercurrent immunoelectrophoresis for *Haemophilus influenzae* and *Streptococcus pneumoniae*.
   (i) RF and autoantibodies.
4. (a) Appropriate antibiotics.
   (b) Pericardiotomy.

Discussion

This patient presents with most of the classic symptoms and signs of acute pericarditis. These are: fever; pain which can be retrosternal (worse on lying down) but also referred to the neck or shoulder since the lower third of the pericardium is innervated by the phrenic nerve; dyspnoea; cough; paradoxical pulse and pericardial rub. Bacterial infections account for about 30% of cases of acute pericarditis in the UK; the usual organisms are staphylococci, streptococci, pneumococci and *Haemophilus influenzae*. Most frequently it is caused by a spread from a pulmonary septic focus. This is the most likely explanation in this boy. The FBC is highly suggestive of a bacterial infection, and signs in the chest are consistent with right middle lobe consolidation. Secondly, a viral cause is possible, and coxsackieviruses are most frequently isolated. This used to be labelled idiopathic or benign acute pericarditis and accounts for a further 30% of cases of acute pericarditis. Other viruses such as echovirus, adenovirus and EBV have been isolated.

Tuberculosis as a cause of acute pericarditis is rare in children, except in the tropics, where it should always be kept in mind. It usually spreads from hilar nodes or a lesion in the lung and this should be considered in this patient.

Rheumatoid disease, SLE, malignancy: for example leukaemic or lymphomatous infiltration of the heart, rheumatic fever and post-pericardiotomy syndrome are the other main causes of acute pericarditis. These are particularly unlikely here, because of the lack of accompanying symptoms and signs of the diseases, and the acute nature of this illness.

Investigations are self-evident: ECG to show concave ST wave elevation and possibly T wave inversion; chest X-ray to show cardiomegaly with loss of the cardiac outline to a more spherical shape; X-ray screening may show the cardiac contour differentiated within the spherical shape; echocardiogram (a reliable, non-invasive method of confirming the presence of a pericardial effusion); pericardial tap–mandatory in order to obtain fluid for microscopy and culture; blood culture in case of a septicaemia, which is common in cases of bacterial aetiology. Other investigations mentioned are not urgent.

Active treatment with appropriate antibiotics is indicated in this child. Purulent pericarditis is usually treated with surgical drainage; fatalities are almost always due to failure to perform a surgical pericardiotomy.

Further reading

Benzing, O. and Kaplan, S. (1953). Purulent pericarditis. *American Journal of Diseases of Children*, **106**, 289.

Jordan, S. C. and Scott, O. (1989). *Heart Disease in Paediatrics*, pp. 313–16. (London; Butterworths)

Marks, M. I. (1985). *Pediatric Infectious Diseases for the Practitioner*, pp. 710–14. (New York; Springer-Verlag)

Case 65

Answers

1. (a) Marfan's syndrome.
   (b) Homocystinuria.
2. (a) Increased urinary excretion of hydroxyproline in Marfan's syndrome.
   (b) Increased urinary excretion of homocystine.

Discussion

Five of the children attend the school yet only two are singled out for unwelcome attention. This suggests that there are visible abnormalities which may be inherited. The child is abnormally tall and has pectus excavatum. He also has ocular abnormalities, including an episode of acute glaucoma and now retinal detachment. Two diseases which explain these findings are Marfan's syndrome and homocystinuria. Other differential diagnoses of excess height such as Kleinfelter's syndrome and juvenile acromegaly do not explain all the stigmata, especially the eye signs.

Marfan's syndrome is an autosomal dominant inherited disease with an incidence of 2–3 per 200 000 population. The biochemical abnormality involves mucopolysaccharide metabolism causing defects in connective tissue and excess urinary excretion of hydroxyproline.

The earliest sign may be the upward dislocation of the lens, which can occur congenitally. Lens dislocation in homocystinuria is downward and is never present at birth. Other ocular changes common to both diseases are myopia, glaucoma and retinal detachment.

Skeletal abnormalities include excess height, arachnodactyly, chest deformity, often pectus excavatum and spinal problems which may include kyphoscoliosis, hemivertebrae, vertebral fusion and spina bifida. The joints are hyperextensible–Steinberg's sign, extension of the opposed thumb past the ulnar border of the hand, is positive. The skeletal changes are thought to be due to generalized endochondral hyperplasia.

Severe cardiothoracic abnormalities may occur. The aorta and pulmonary artery may dilate with subsequent aneurysm formation and dissection. Valvular abnormalities include aortic and mitral incompetence. Congenital heart disease is rare, but has been described in association with Marfan's syndrome. Lesions described include Fallot's tetralogy, patent ductus arteriosus, stenosis of the aortic isthmus and ventricular septal defect.

Homocystinuria is a recessively inherited abnormality of amino acid metabolism due to a deficiency of cystathionine synthetase. Homocystine is an important intermediate in methionine metabolism which is included in protein synthesis. This may explain the connective tissue malfunction. Clinical features are manifest in three main areas: connective tissue, thrombotic phenomena and neuropsychiatric disturbances. A malar flush is common and telangiectasis may occur at the edge of scar tissue. The hair is fair and sparse. Ocular changes include cataracts in addition to those already mentioned. Skeletal abnormalities include excess height with increased span, kyphoscoliosis and pectus excavatum. Generalized osteoporosis occurs, which predisposes to spontaneous fractures. Joint mobility is reduced and Steinberg's sign is negative, in contradistinction to Marfan's syndrome.

Thrombotic episodes occur in virtually all affected patients and no vessel is immune. Angina pectoris or sudden death may occur from involvement of the coronary arteries. Repeated cerebral thrombosis is a factor in the neuropsychiatric manifestations. Only 50% of sufferers have normal intelligence. It has been suggested that a schizoid personality is common in this disease.

Two varieties of homocystinuria are recognized, one pyridoxine-sensitive, the other pyridoxine-resistant. The former may respond to pharmaceutical doses of vitamin B_6. Both may be treated, with varying success, with a diet low in methionine but with added cystine.

Further reading

Pierpoint, M. E. M. and Moller J. H. (1989). Cardiac manifestations of systemic disease. In *Moss' Heart Disease in Infants, Children and Adolescents*, 4th edn, Ed. by F. H. Adams, G. C. Emmanouilides and T. A. Riemenschneider, pp. 792–6. (Baltimore; Williams & Wilkins)

Carson, N. A. J. (1982). Homocystinuria: clinical and biochemical heterogeneity. In *Inborn Errors of Metabolism in Humans*, Ed. by F. Cockburn and R. Gitzelman, pp. 53–64. (Lancaster; MTP Press)

Case 66

Answers

1. Isoimmune thrombocytopenia.
2. (a) Maternal blood count, particularly platelets.
   (b) Platelet antibody studies on mother and child, particularly against father's platelets.
3. (a) Intravenous immunoglobin.
   (b) Platelet transfusions, especially with mother's washed platelets.
   (c) Exchange transfusion.

Discussion

There are several causes of thrombocytopenia in a neonate, such as, maternal idiopathic thrombocytopenic purpura (ITP), intrauterine infection, DIC, sepsis, congenital thrombocytopenia or leukaemia, and maternal drug ingestion. All of these may occur in one child, but three successive children with thrombocytopenia suggests a common process, the most likely being isoimmune thrombocytopenia or undiagnosed maternal ITP. The latter should be excluded by a maternal platelet count. It is most unusual to find significant neonatal thrombocytopenia without marked maternal thrombocytopenia, i.e. a platelet count $<100 \times 10^9$/litre, unless there is a past history of splenectomy and this should always be sought. This was not the situation in this case.

In isoimmune thrombocytopenia a mechanism similar to rhesus disease of the newborn operates in which mother develops antibodies to a factor on father's platelets; the usual antibody is anti-Pl Al. Some 98% of mothers are Pl Al-positive, 2% of mothers are Pl Al-negative, hence this 2% may develop anti-Pl Al antibodies. Diagnosis is confirmed by the demonstration that maternal serum contains anti-Pl Al antibodies, usually by means of immunofluorescence or enzyme-linked immunoassay techniques. Maternal platelet count is normal.

Treatment must aim to tide the baby over the vulnerable period of thrombocytopenia when the main danger is intra-cerebral haemorrhage, and secondly to reduce the amount of antibody. Platelet transfusions may be helpful, but these have a short life, and will have to be repeated as the platelets are destroyed by the antibodies present. Thus mother's washed platelets resuspended in compatible plasma are the most logical source to use. Intravenous immunoglobulin given for 3–5 days has been found to be effective in increasing the platelet count, and should be the first line of treatment. Thirdly, exchange transfusion with fresh blood can be employed as in rhesus incompatibility. Previously steroids were used in this condition but are not as useful as in thrombocytopenia secondary to maternal ITP.

If there is any diagnostic doubt then other investigations should be done, i.e. TORCH and clotting screens, blood culture and bone marrow aspiration. Very rare causes of neonatal thrombocytopenia are maternal SLE, Wiskott–Aldrich syndrome or Fanconi/absent radii syndromes.

Further reading

Levene, M. I., Tudehope, D. and Thearle, J. (1987). *Essentials of Neonatal Medicine*, pp. 245–50. (Oxford; Blackwell Scientific Publications)

Napier, J. A. F. (1987). *Blood Transfusion Therapy*, pp. 248–50. (Chichester; John Wiley)

Robertson, N. R. C. (1986). *Textbook of Neonatology*, pp. 444–6. (Edinburgh; Churchill Livingstone)

Case 67

Answers

1. Ectopic ureter opening distal to the bladder.

2. (a) IVP.
   (b) Micturating cystourethrogram (MCU).
   (c) Ultrasound.
   (d) Aortogram.

Discussion

The history of this child is classic of a low-placed ectopic ureter either in the lower urethra, vestibule or vagina. There is persistent dampness despite normal micturition at normal intervals. There are several other causes of persistent dribbling including neurogenic bladder, ectopic ureterocele causing infravesical obstruction, and posterior urethral valves, but none is accompanied by normal micturition. Certain diagnosis can, however, be difficult. An IVP will demonstrate a non-opacified upper pole of the affected kidney, but as the renal remnant is often unable to concentrate any dye, the ureter may not be delineated. A large, tortuous ureter may be demonstrated by ultrasound, but ultrasonography is an unreliable investigation for ureteric abnormalities. Occasionally a renal arteriogram or an aortogram can be used. It may be possible to detect a urethral opening on urethroscopy, but high vaginal openings are notoriously difficult to find. A micturating cystourethrogram may demonstrate reflux into the ectopic ureter if the opening is in the bladder or upper urethra. If all else fails, an exploratory operation is indicated.

Treatment is by heminephroureterectomy or nephroureterectomy as the renal tissue drained by the ectopic ureter usually has poor or no function. Re-implantation has little to offer, therefore. The complete length of the ureter should be removed, except in boys if there is involvement of the vas deferens and seminal vesicle.

Accessory ureteric buds arise cranial to the normal buds and, therefore, drain the upper renal moiety; however, the distal opening is always lower than that of the normal ureter and may involve the bladder neck, posterior urethra, wolffian or müllerian duct derivatives. If both ureters from a kidney are ectopic, that draining the upper moiety still drains to a lower point than the other. Ectopic ureters are subject to dilatation and reflux except for those opening into the trigone where there appears to be sufficient muscular tone to prevent reflux.

The mode of presentation depends on the positioning of the ureter and the sex of the child. The commonest ectopic position in females is in the bladder neck area. Incontinence is not a feature and presentation is severe, persistent or recurrent pyuria.

If the opening is lower, infection is far less common and, characteristically, the child presents with persistent dribbling incontinence punctuated by normal micturition. Occasionally the child may be dry at night, probably due to a reservoir effect of the dilated ureter. Rarely, the child may have been completely dry before the onset of symptoms. This usually occurs when the ectopic opening is in the lower urethra; the musculature maintains continence until the ureter becomes dilated.

In males, the ectopic ureter may join the posterior urethra, ejaculatory duct or vas deferens. Incontinence is rarer than in the female, the presenting complaints commonly being severe pyuria or epididymitis. Often there is a single ectopic ureter draining the whole kidney which is itself dysplastic or ectopic. Diagnosis and treatment are as outlined above.

Further reading

Innes-Williams, D. and Johnston, J. H. (eds) (1982). *Paediatric Urology*, 2nd edn, pp. 167–87. (London; Butterworths)

Rickwood, A. M. K. (1990). Indications for investigation of the urinary tract in the newborn. In *Neonatal Surgery*, 3rd edn, Ed. by J. Lister and I. M. Irving, pp. 649–54. (London; Butterworths)

Case 68

Answers

1. (a) *Mycoplasma pneumoniae* antibody titres.
   (b) *M. pneumoniae* complement fixation test.
   (c) Cold agglutinin titre.
   (d) Viral antibodies.
   (e) Psittacosis, Q fever and legionella complement fixation titres.
2. (a) Erythromycin.
   (b) Tetracycline.

Discussion

This case history gives away the diagnosis by the classic history of *Mycoplasma pneumoniae* infection. On reading the case history initially one thinks of tuberculosis, but the negative Mantoux test result and lack of lymphocytosis in the peripheral blood and pleural fluid make this diagnosis most unlikely. An atypical pneumonia in which there are clinical signs of lower respiratory tract infection associated with respiratory symptoms, but lack of response to the usual antibiotics employed such as amoxycillin, is usually caused by *M. pneumoniae* but other organisms that should be considered are viruses, especially the adenovirus, *Chlamydia psittaci*, i.e. psittacosis, and *Coxiella burnetii*, i.e. Q fever pneumonia.

Mycoplasma infections are most frequent in school-age children. However, in children under 5, when screened, many asymptomatic infections have been found. Pneumonic disease in the older age groups may be an expression of increasing host immune response to the organism, and many of the complications may result through immunological mechanisms. The incubation period is about 12–14 days. The first symptoms are flu-like, with headache, fever, chills, malaise and anorexia followed by a sore throat and dry cough.

Other symptoms include nasal discharge, vomiting, abdominal pain, earache, and non-specific skin rashes. Mucoid sputum may be produced later, and when seen in hospital a large number of patients have failed to respond to antibiotics.

Physical signs are very variable. Fever is usual, but chest signs can be lobar, unilateral, bilateral or generalized, and generally consist both of crepitations and, less frequently, of rhonchi. Occasionally a pleural effusion may be present. Pharyngeal oedema, skin rashes, tender cervical lymph nodes, otitis media and conjunctivitis may also be present.

The chest X-ray is also variable with either a lobar or multifocal consolidation. Quite frequently the chest X-ray changes are mild in comparison with the physical findings and vice versa. If decubitus views are taken, pleural effusions are found in up to a quarter of cases. They are exudates, with no organisms on Gram's stain or culture, but with WBC from 5 to 6000×10^9/litre. The peripheral WBC is usually normal with an absolute neutrophilia, as in this case. Cold agglutinins occur in about 50% of cases but are less common in children than adults. If present with a respiratory infection, it is highly suggestive of mycoplasma, although cold agglutinins are also present in infectious mononucleosis, adenovirus and other infections. There is a simple cold agglutinin screening test which can be done at the bedside. This consists of mixing 50:50 blood and citrate together in a prothrombin tube, and placing it in a deep-freezer compartment for a few minutes. On removal obvious agglutination can be seen on the wall of the tube if the test is positive and disappears on warming. Confirmation with antibody titres done by indirect immunofluorescence is a prolonged method; complement fixation titres on acute and convalescent serum showing a fourfold rise or more, or a single titre of 1:64, is highly suggestive; and lastly isolation of *M. pneumoniae* from sputum is possible but difficult.

Differential diagnosis from psittacosis, which may present in a very similar fashion to mycoplasma with diffuse or patchy chest X-ray changes, should be made with rise in complement-fixing antibodies, isolation of the chlamydial organism if possible and a history of exposure to birds. Q fever principally affects the lungs and should be looked for by a rise in antibody titre, but complement fixing or agglutination tests are more reliable. Legionnaire's disease should be considered in the differential diagnosis of severe lobar pneumonia.

Viral infections may be diagnosed by increase in specific antibody titres on paired serum samples approximately 2 weeks apart, if these are available.

Reported complications of mycoplasma infections are many and variable. These include bullous myringitis, Stevens–Johnson syndrome, adult respiratory distress syndrome, haemolytic anaemia, myocarditis, Guillain–Barré syndrome, poliomyelitis-like syndrome, meningitis, arthritis, glomerulonephritis, genital disease and sterility.

Treatment is usually with erythromycin in children but tetracycline may be used in children over 12 years when the danger of permanently staining the teeth is over.

Further reading

Fernald, G. W. *et al.* (1979). Respiratory infections due to *Mycoplasma pneumoniae* in infants and children. *Pediatrics*, **55**, 327–35.

Lane, D. J. (1979). Pneumonia. *Medicine*, **23**, 1177–82.

Levine, D. P. and Lerner, A. M. (1978). The clinical spectrum of *Mycoplasma pneumoniae* infection. *Medical Clinics of North America*, **62**, 961–78.

McFarlane, J. T. *et al.* (1979). Rapid diagnosis of *Mycoplasma pneumoniae* infection; a reminder. *British Medical Journal*, **i**, 124.

Pumarola, A., *et al.* (1979). *Mycoplasma pneumoniae* infections. *Paediatrician*, **8**, 56–64.

Stevens, D. *et al.* (1978). *Mycoplasma pneumoniae* infections in children. *Archives of Disease in Childhood*, **53**, 38–42.

Case 69

Answers

1. (a) Establishment of an airway.
   (b) Intravenous antibiotics.
2. (a) Blood gases.
   (b) Blood cultures.
   (c) Lateral X-ray of neck.
   (d) Bacterial throat swabs.

Discussion

This child presents clinically with acute epiglottitis which is commonly caused by *Haemophilus influenzae* type B. The history is short and he presents as a toxic, pyrexial child with respiratory embarrassment, cyanosis from hypoxia and restlessness from hypercapnia. The immediate action is to ensure the patency of the airway. Acute epiglottitis is a rapidly progressive, potentially lethal disease, so speed in establishing an airway is of paramount importance. The child may be intubated by an experienced anaesthetist, preferably with an ENT surgeon in attendance, or an elective tracheostomy can be performed. As an emergency nebulized adrenaline can be used to reduce glottic swelling whilst awaiting intubation. The child is then given humidified air to breathe. Once the airway is established the appropriate intravenous antibiotics are given: 15% of *H. influenzae* are resistant to ampicillin. Blood gases are taken to assess oxygenation. There is still debate as to the efficacy of steroids in reducing tissue oedema.

Acute epiglottitis is the most likely diagnosis and may be confirmed by appropriate investigation. However, other diagnoses should be considered.

Viral infection of the respiratory tree–such as acute laryngitis, laryngotracheitis or laryngotracheobronchitis–usually has a longer history, but laryngotracheobronchitis may present acutely and, if the oedema extends distally, the respiratory embarrassment may not be relieved by intubation. Implicated viruses are parainfluenza, echoviruses, respiratory syncytial virus and coxsackie viruses. At laryngoscopy the epiglottis is normal, but there is marked oedema distally. Treatment is also by intubation if indicated or by humidified air. Antibiotics are not indicated. Occasionally *H. influenzae* can cause laryngotracheobronchitis. If this is considered, appropriate antibiotics should be started. Inhaled foreign bodies may impact in the glottis and cause immediate stridor which is worsened by subsequent oedema or mucosal haemorrhage. This would not, however, produce such a high pyrexia. Differentiation is often possible on lateral neck X-ray.

Angioneurotic oedema may present rapidly after an inhaled or ingested allergen. No rash indicating urticaria was noted, although oedema may occur without a peripheral rash. At laryngoscopy the tissues are pale and oedematous rather than brilliant red in the infective states. Treatment is with subcutaneous adrenaline or intravenous hydrocortisone and antihistamines.

Further reading

Boon, A. W. (1987). Upper airways obstruction. In *Paediatric Emergencies*, 2nd edn, Ed. by J. A. Black, pp. 207–8. (London; Butterworths)

Phelan, P. D. Landau, L. I. and Olinsky, A. (eds) (1990). Clinical patterns of acute respiratory infections. In *Respiratory Illness in Children*, pp. 60–2. (Oxford; Blackwell Scientific Publications)

Case 70

Answers

1. ECG.
2. Aortic stenosis.
3. (a) Echocardiography with Doppler studies.
   (b) Cardiac catheterization.

Discussion

This previously healthy child presents with a sudden transient loss of consciousness with no neurological sequelae. This argues against a toxic or infective encephalopathy. The immediate thought, therefore, may be of a simple faint. The weather was hot, the episode short, the blood pressure marginally low and there were no sequelae. However, a diastolic murmur is pathological and combined with a systolic murmur, a soft second sound and a marginally low blood pressure, suggests aortic stenosis with incompetence. An ECG would show left ventricular hypertrophy with large R and S waves in the left and right leads, respectively. Left-sided strain is indicated by ST depression with or without T wave inversion over the left chest leads.

Echocardigraphy is a useful non-invasive technique for viewing the aortic valve and outflow tract. Colour Doppler now allows accurate assesment of the transvalvular pressure without resorting to the more invasive catheterization.

Aortic stenosis constitutes 5% of cardiac malformations and is three times more prevalent in males than females. The obstruction may be supravalvular, valvular or subvalvular. Valvular may be either fused cusps or an abnormal bicuspid valve, as in this child. Subvalvular may be either discrete, such as a fibrous ring, or a diffuse obstructive cardiomyopathy–hypertrophic obstructive cardiomyopathy (HOCM).

Many children are symptomless, even with moderately severe stenosis. Others may have dyspnoea on exertion or cerebral hypoxia causing loss of consciousness. Aortic stenosis is always quoted as one of the causes of childhood angina, but chest pain occurs in the minority of cases.

Examination may reveal jerky pulses in HOCM or an anacrotic pulse in the other types. The systolic blood pressure may be reduced, but often not strikingly so. The second heart sound may be soft or have reversed splitting. The ejection systolic murmur may be heard at the apex, base or left sternal edge. An early systolic click may be heard at the apex. In severe disease a double atrial beat may be felt.

Surgery is indicated by the presence of chest pain, loss of consciousness, ST depression on an ECG and a pressure gradient in excess of 55 mmHg across the stenotic valve.

Sadly, this congenital anomaly is a cause of sudden death and it is extremely difficult to define the 'at-risk' population. There is usually no family history, except occasionally in HOCM which can have an autosomal dominant inheritance, and the children are often symptomless.

Further reading

Friedman, W. F. (1989). Aortic stenosis. In *Moss' Heart Disease in Infants, Children and Adolescents*, 4th edn, Ed. by F. H. Adams, G. C. Emmanouilides and T. A. Riemenschneider, pp. 224–40. (Baltimore; Williams & Wilkins)

Case 71

Answers

1. Pulmonary atresia with an intact ventricular septum.
2. (a) Echocardiography.
   (b) Cardiac catheterization.

Discussion

This infant has a ductus arteriosus-dependent cyanotic cardiac lesion. The indomethacin infusion caused a partial closure of the duct. This caused a deep cyanosis which was reversed by prostaglandin E. Having partially closed the duct, the wisdom of then placing the child in oxygen, with the possibility of further ductal closure, is debatable. The ventricular septum must be intact and there must also be a right-to-left shunt. If there was a left-to-right shunt, one would expect right ventricle dominance on the ECG and plethoric lung fields. The most common possibilities, therefore, are transposition of the great vessels and tricuspid or pulmonary atresia, or pin-hole stenosis.

The chest X-ray was reported as oligaemic, which is against transposition; also the adult pattern is not typical of a transposition ECG. A single second sound may be heard, however.

The findings are also not entirely consistent with tricuspid atresia. The chest X-ray findings can be similar, the second sound may be single, but the ECG classically displays a left axis deviation. The most likely diagnosis is, therefore, pulmonary atresia or severe stenosis, with an intact ventricular septum.

Pulmonary atresia is rare, accounting for only 1% of congenital cardiac lesions. The atresia is usually valvular only but may occasionally be infundibular. There are two main varieties. The more common (80–85%) have a small right ventricle associated with a hypoplastic tricuspid valve; the rest have a normal or large right ventricle, often associated with tricuspid incompetence. Either type may have an intact or perforated ventricular septum. If the septum is intact, pulmonary flow is via a patent ductus arteriosus and the bronchial vessels.

Pulmonary atresia has developmental consequences. The aorta does not taper smoothly and does not have an isthmal narrowing or post-ductal dilatation, the pulmonary artery is very small and there is a reversal of flow in the ductus arteriosus. If the ductus is small, marked cyanosis occurs; if large, cyanosis may be absent. On auscultation, the first heart sound is invariably single if the right ventricle and tricuspid valve are small. There may be a soft mid systolic murmur from the ductus arteriosus. With a large right ventricle, the first sound may also be single and the systolic murmurs are consequent on the anatomy of the tricuspid valve. The second heart sound is obviously single. The ECG may be the key to diagnosis as the combination of cyanosis with left ventricular dominance is highly suggestive of pulmonary atresia. There is a normal right-sided axis.

The cardiac silhouette is usually normal in the neonatal period, but the left ventricle and right atrium rapidly enlarge, as does the aorta.

The echocardiogram is useful for determining chamber and vessel size; confirmation can be obtained by cardiac catheterization or by cardiac angiography.

The prognosis is poor–up to 50% of infants die within the first month of life. Surgical treatment is possible and approaches include the formation of a pulmonary systemic anastomosis, reconstruction of the pulmonary outflow tract and the construction of an external conduit from the right atrium or ventricle to the pulmonary artery.

Further reading

Marvin, W. J. and Mahoney, L. T. (1989). Pulmonary atresia with intact ventricular septum. In *Moss' Heart Disease in Infancy, Children and Adolescents*, 4th edn, Ed. by F. H. Adams, G. C. Emmanouilides and T. A. Riemenschneider, pp. 338–46. (Baltimore; Williams & Wilkins)

Case 72

Answers

1. (a) Blood sugar.
   (b) EEG.
2. (a) Pseudofits.
   (b) Hysteria.
   (c) Münchausen by proxy.
3. Child and family therapy.

Discussion

This child had experienced hypoglycaemic episodes following discharge. However, mimicry of simple absences would be an unusual manifestation of hypoglycaemia; it is virtually inconceivable that hypoglycaemia would be the cause of prolonged absences. She is, however, diabetic: knowledge of her glycaemic status is therefore mandatory.

One simple absence was witnessed in Outpatients. The description and the witnessed episode appeared sufficiently impressive for drug therapy to be instituted. As one episode was witnessed the history was not fabricated and Münchausen syndrome by proxy is unlikely as either the history is fabricated or induction of fits normally results in tonic clonic fits. The change in length of fit to 10 min militates against these being simple absences. Atypical absence seizures or Lennox–Gestaut syndrome present ealier in life (1–3 years) and are normally associated with mental retardation.

Sammie's EEG was normal, although a normal EEG does not exclude epilepsy, as many children have non-paroxysmal recordings. It is unlikely that interpretation was a problem; the EEG may still have been maturing at her age, both with respect to fast beta activity and slower theta and delta rhythms. The characteristic spike and wave activity is obvious in the paediatric EEG.

The possibility of pseudoseizures or hysteria manifest as pseudoseizures is raised. This child had experienced several major life events recently–the divorce of her parents, a new school, her mother's remarriage and the onset of diabetes. Hysteria is an unconscious strategy adopted to cope with or avoid anxiety, the primary gain perpetuated by the secondary aim of increased attention. It is perhaps not surprising that this girl took such refuge to cope with the effect of the several negative life events.

Hysterical reactions in older children and adolescents frequently manifest as movement disorders, loss of movement of a limb or limbs, seizures or loss of sight or speech. It can be difficult, however, to differentiate between the unconscious or deliberate adoption of the disability. Once the child or adolescent is 'sick' a way out of the 'sickness' must be found which avoids the child losing face in his or her domestic environment, or a cure will not be affected. Fortunately, the majority of children respond well to firm reassurance. Those who do not can be difficult to treat.

Another possible diagnosis is Münchausen's syndrome or Münchausen's syndrome by proxy. In all children with bizarre inexplicable neurological disorders, a toxicological cause should be considered. Sammie was arguably too old for the proxy syndrome; case reports of poisoning or the deliberate administration of inappropriate medication have tended to be in younger children. It is difficult to think of a medication which would induce a statue like stance for 5 min or longer, followed by normal behaviour. Hysterical conversion thus remains the favoured diagnosis.

Further reading

Hersov, L. (1985). Emotional disorders. In *Child and Adolescent Psychiatry. Modern Approaches*, 2nd edn, Ed. by M. Rutter and L. Hersov, pp. 373–5. (Oxford; Blackwell Scientific Publications)

Steinberg, D. (ed.) (1983). *The Clinical Psychiatry of Adolescence*, pp. 178–80. (Chichester; John Wiley)

Case 73

Answers

1. (a) HIV antigen.
   (b) HIV antibody.
   (c) Lymphocyte typing, CD4, CD8.
   (d) TORCH antibodies.

    (e) Stool culture for *Cryptosporidium*.
2. (a) HIV infection.
    (b) Intrauterine infection.
3. Lymphocytic interstitial pneumonitis.

Discussion

This infant presents with a generalized systemic disturbance, pyrexia, tachypnoea, generalized reticuloendothelial activation, failure to thrive and diarrhoea. The initial diagnosis of ALL was neither substantiated peripherally nor on marrow aspiration. This concatenation of signs is non-specific; it could be that the failure to thrive and repeated diarrhoea were related to the domestic environment and a further infection precipitated consultation. However, generalized lymphadenopathy is difficult to explain; if related to the presence of dogs in the squat, intense peripheral eosinophilia would be present with systemic *Toxocara canis*.

An intrauterine infection could explain the lymphadenopathy. It is likely that this would have been a third-trimester infection, yet no mention of the classical triad of jaundice, hepatomegaly and thrombocytopenia was made at birth. Generally the signs disappear within the first few months of life, the jaundice usually fading in 3–4 weeks, although if the hepatitis is severe, jaundice may persist for several months. Hepatosplenomegaly may persist for many months, but is not accompanied by persisting lymphadenopathy. The neurological prognosis depends on the gestational age at infection and the infecting organism. Neurological impairment is common in CMV infection, whereas third-trimester rubella infection often has a good neurological prognosis, although there is a high mortality rate if severe thrombocytopenia persists.

There is a hint that this infant may be immunocompromised; he suffered a severe bacterial infection at 8 weeks of life and has had three episodes of gastroenteritis. His father has travelled repeatedly to an area of high risk for HIV infection and despite antibiotic treatment and oral electrolyte solution his signs continue and he has grossly elevated immunoglobulins. In these circumstances HIV infection should be considered. It is important to remember that, at present, parental consent, which should be accompanied by counselling, must be obtained before HIV testing can be undertaken.

The diagnosis of HIV infection in infancy is still difficult. Maternal IgG antibodies pass through the placenta and may persist for up to 18 months of age, although the median is 8 months. Identification of IgM HIV antibodies would suggest active neonatal infection but, as yet, the laboratory techniques are not sufficiently sensitive to allow definitive diagnosis. The same problem is encountered in viral culture and P24-antigen detection. Tests of immune activation such as raised immunoglobulin levels, serum neopterin and β_2-microglobulin levels with a decreasing number of CD4 T cells can be used to predict the progression to AIDS of infants born to HIV-positive mothers. However, again these tests are not widely available and have yet to be standardized. Thus the diagnosis of HIV will only become established if the infant develops clinical AIDS or maternal antibodies are replaced by the infant's own in the second or subsequent year of life.

Vertical transmission is the commonest route of infection in childhood; the introduction of a heat-treated factor VIII has removed the risk of infection in haemophiliacs. The risk of maternal transfer varies enormously from study to study; one factor in this is the lack of homogeneity between the populations studied. Studies report transmission rates which vary from 15 to 60%–the lower rates are reported from Europe, the higher from Africa.

HIV-positive infants are prone to bacterial infections, from which this infant suffered. There is a significant incidence, 20–40%, of lymphocytic interstitial pneumonitis, the most likely cause of this child's tachypnoea. The gastroenteritis could be caused by *Cryptosporidium*; this organism causes about 4% of community-acquired diarrhoea, but can cause persistent and torrential diarrhoea in HIV.

The distinction between HIV, AIDS-related complex (ARC) and AIDS is not so clear as in adults. Failure to thrive is common in uninfected infants from communities with a high incidence of HIV, diarrhoea similarly. If, however, the failure to thrive persists despite adequate treatment of concurrent infection and good nutrition, then it is arguable that this child has ARC and would then fall into a poor prognostic group.

The guidelines for treatment of infantile HIV are still debated. The difficulty in obtaining a precise diagnosis coupled with toxicity of the available drugs makes treatment in those without frank ARC or AIDS controversial, although there is some evidence that early treatment does improve prognosis and delaying treatment may compromise the prognosis.

252

Further reading

Gibb, D. M. (1991). HIV infection in children. *Hospital Update*, **17**, 267–81.

Hira, S. K., Kamanga, J., Bhat, G. J., Mwale, C., Tembo, G., Luo, N. and Perine, P. L. (1989). Perinatal transmission of HIV-1 in Zambia. *British Medical Journal*, **299**, 1250–2.

Mok, J. (1991). HIV infection in children. *British Medical Journal*, **302**, 921–2.

Pizzo, P. A. and Wilfert, C. M. (1990). Treatment considerations for children with human immunodeficiency virus infection. *Pediatric Infectious Diseases*, **9**, 690–9.

Case 74

Answers

1. Lactose intolerance
2. (a) Stool-reducing substances
   (b) Stool pH.

Discussion

This baby presents with what looks at first sight to be a complicated renal or metabolic problem and possibly an infection. The main components are a respiratory compensated metabolic acidosis; hypoglycaemia; hypocalcaemia, which probably resulted from hyperventilation, hence a low $P\mathrm{co}_2$; and lastly, dehydration.

The history is one of difficulties with feeding right from the start, even with breast milk. The baby apparently improved rapidly on intravenous fluids, although the urea and electrolytes did not return to normal, but it was not until milk was restarted that her clinical condition deteriorated again with increasing acidosis, dehydration and hypocalcaemia. Investigations for abnormalities of the pyruvate and urea cycles, i.e. ammonia and lactate levels, were normal–it is common to get borderline levels possibly due to dehydration; if they are significant, the levels should be markedly above the normal range. Secondly the clinical condition of a baby with a complicated metabolic problem does not improve dramatically overnight with intravenous fluids–it takes longer.

At this stage we should look at other possibilities, such as infection, but cultures were negative; congenital infection does not explain the problem as there is no hepatosplenomegaly or thrombocytopenia. Renal problems are a distinct possibility but renal ultrasound is normal, excluding a structural abnormality. Onset here is very early; this can occur in the infantile forms of RTA, but the clinical picture is usually one of hyperchloraemic metabolic acidosis in the absence of an overall decrease in renal function. Distal RTA inherited as an autosomal recessive usually has the acidifying defect present at birth, i.e. inability to maintain H^+ gradient in the distal tubule and collecting duct. Early presentation is rare, but in this case a urinary pH of less than 6.0 in the face of severe acidosis would have excluded the diagnosis. The usual presentation of distal RTA is with failure to thrive and polyuria from early infancy. Proximal RTA usually presents in the first 18 months with growth failure and vomiting.

Having looked at the various possibilities, one must come back to the history–problems with milk, even breast milk, with diarrhoea, tense abdomen and irritability associated with acidosis. Lactose intolerance results in fermentation of lactose in the bowel lumen forming frothy, watery, acidic stools. It would appear that such an acid load in the infant's immature bowel is readily absorbed, hence the metabolic upset, plus dehydration from fluid loss. Frequently the diarrhoea is not as prominent a sign as would appear from the metabolic upset and is therefore disregarded. In this case stool pH was 5.5 and faecal-reducing substances were heavily positive.

There are three types of lactose intolerance which present in infancy: primary congenital alactasia, congenital lactose intolerance and secondary lactose deficiency. In primary congenital alactasia diarrhoea occurs from birth and ceases when lactose is removed from the diet. Lactose intolerance continues into childhood; lactase activity is virtually absent on jejunal biopsy, where other disaccharidase activities are normal. This form is rare.

In congenital lactose intolerance infants characteristically have vomiting, diarrhoea and failure to thrive associated with large amounts of lactose and sometimes sucrose excreted in the urine. This syndrome remains a mystery. Outcome can be fatal, but lactase levels are usually normal and the diarrhoea is not of the severity or type seen in lactase deficiency.

Lastly, secondary lactase deficiency follows an episode of gastroenteritis. This is usually temporary while the intestinal mucosa recovers its normal architecture.

In this case the early onset with severe diarrhoea and constitutional upset make congenital alactasia the most likely diagnosis.

Further reading

Anderson, C. M. (1971). Disorders of carbohydrate absorption in childhood. *Journal of Clinical Pathology*, **24** (suppl. 5), 14–21.

Walker-Smith, J. (1988). *Diseases of the Small Intestine in Childhood*, 3rd edn, pp. 315–22. (London; Butterworths)

Case 75

Answers

1. Bronchiectasis or chronic suppurative lung disease.
2. (a) Cilial dyskinesia/immotile cilia syndrome.
   (b) Kartagener's syndrome.
   (c) Congenital pneumonia with imcomplete resolution.
   (d) Sequestered lower lobe.
3. (a) Bronchogram.
   (b) Nasal mucosa brushings for cilial investigations.
   (c) Ventilation/perfusion scan.
   (d) Pulmonary angiography.

Discussion

This 6-year-old girl has the symptoms and signs of chronic suppurative lung disease–extensive consolidation on X-ray, clubbing, infected sputum production and recurrent infective episodes. There are many possible causes which fit into four main categories: acute pneumonia, recurrent lower respiratory tract infection, underlying chronic disease or structural abnormality of the lung. Several diagnoses have been ruled out by the investigations provided.

Looking first at underlying chronic disease, the most common is cystic fibrosis, but this girl is not failing to thrive and the sweat test is normal; immune deficiency is unlikely in view of the onset at age 5 years of recurrent infection, the lack of other types of infection, normal immunoglobulins, normal numbers of neutrophils and lymphocytes; alpha, antitrypsin deficiency has been ruled out with a protein electrophoresis showing a normal alpha band, also there was no history of neonatal jaundice.

In an otherwise normal child a severe episode of bacterial or viral pneumonia may result in bronchiectasis; measles and pertussis have frequently been implicated in the past. This child had neonatal pneumonia and appears to have had problems on and off ever since. If vigorous treatment is not given at the time and the lung re-expanded, only partial recovery occurs, predisposing to further infection and damage. A ventilation/perfusion scan may be helpful in this instance.

Recurrent lower respiratory tract infection may lead to bronchiectasis, for example, recurrent aspiration, which seems unlikely here since there is no suggestive history of cough on feeding and problems would have arisen at a much earlier age; or following inhalation of a foreign body with incomplete resolution or bronchial damage. Finally, chronic sinusitis occasionally results in repeated chest infections even in a child of this age. These problems may masquerade as asthma, hence any infant or young child who has frequent or severe attacks should have a more detailed investigation including barium swallow.

Structural abnormality of the lungs can take various forms. Lobar sequestration occurs twice as commonly in the left as the right lower lobe. Typically there are persistent cystic changes on chest X-ray and the ventilation/perfusion scan shows poor ventilation and no perfusion because of the systemic blood supply. Direct vascular imaging with angiography is undertaken to confirm the lesion. Disorders of the cilia take various forms, the most classical being Kartagener's syndrome which is associated with situs inversus (dextrocardia is of particular note) and chronic sinusitis. Only about 50% of patients presenting with ciliary defect actually have classical Kartagener's syndrome. Diagnosis is made by obtaining cilia via a special nasal brushing technique and examining them immediately for motility by a photometric method, and under the electron microscope.

It was thought that this child had ciliary dyskinesia because of the previous sinusitis and deafness, even though this was not conductive in aetiology. However, investigations were all negative, leaving a congenital pneumonia as the probable cause of her bronchiectasis. A bronchogram should be performed to delineate the extent of the bronchiectasis. If it is localized to a particular segment or lobe, as in this case, but infection is spilling over to the rest of the lung, then surgery should be considered.

Further reading

Buchdahl, R. M. *et al.* (1988). Ciliary abnormalities in respiratory disease. *Archives of Disease in Childhood*, **63**, 238–43.

Dinwiddie, R. (1990). *The Diagnosis and Management of Paediatric Respiratory Disease*, pp. 67; 105; 118–19; 129–31. (Edinburgh; Churchill Livingstone)

Simpson, H. and Mok, J. Y. Q. (1985). Outcome of respiratory disease in childhood. In *Neonatal Pediatric and Respiratory Medicine*, Ed. by A. D. Milner and R. J. Martin, pp. 211–29. (London; Butterworths)

Case 76

Answer

1. Infective endocarditis.

Discussion

The most striking feature here is the unremarkable history in association with surprising signs and investigations. In particular the marked anaemia, mild thrombocytopenia and raised C-reactive protein should make one consider the positive blood culture seriously. *Moraxella* spp. is one of the genus *Neisseria*, a Gram-negative diplococcus usually associated with conjunctivitis. It is a very infrequent contaminant in blood culture, especially when grown from both bottles. Whenever in doubt, blood cultures should be repeated and a microbiologist consulted.

Many children have borderline anaemia–Hb approximately 10 g/100 ml–at the age of 1 year. Below this there is often a pathological reason. The possible causes are a haemoglobinopathy, aplasia secondary to a parvovirus infection and haemolytic anaemia, a chronic infection, acute bleed, cows' milk protein intolerance, iron deficiency or a malignancy. The normal MCV and MCHC make a haemoglobinopathy and iron deficiency unlikely; cows' milk protein intolerance can present with an iron-deficiency picture from chronic loss of blood in the gastrointestinal tract. The reticulocyte count of 2.4% is too high for aplasia, too low for a haemolytic anaemia or following an acute bleed.

The normochromic normocytic anaemia with slightly depressed marrow, i.e. mild thrombocytopenia and low reticulocyte count in response to severe anaemia, would fit with infection or malignancy, but the mild leukocytosis with the clinical features of poor feeding and weight gain, temperature and splenomegaly all support chronic infection. All systems should be investigated– renal tract, chest, head, bones and joints, gastrointestinal tract and heart. The history and examination suggest infective endo- carditis, even though it is very unusual under the age of 2 years and in a child with no previous history of heart murmur. This infant had never been ill, gained weight satisfactorily and was therefore only examined by a doctor at the postnatal and 6-week examinations. Heart murmurs can easily be missed or thought insignificant.

The initial heart murmur could be put down to a flow murmur from a hyperdynamic circulation secondary to anaemia, but this murmur persisted after transfusion. This, together with splenome- galy, RBCs in the urine, the initial improvement after antibiotics and transfusion, plus subsequent collapse, make infective endo- carditis very likely.

Echocardiogram should be done to look for vegetations and any other sites for infection ruled out. The mild haematuria would be consistent with urinary tract infection or glomerulonephritis, but there were no casts or albuminuria.

Infective endocarditis may occur in any congenital heart lesion, particularly ventricular septal defect, patent ductus arteriosus, coarctation, mitral and aortic valves and infrequently on an iso- lated pulmonary stenosis but never on a secundum atrial septal defect. The vegetations tend to grow at a point where the blood stream impinges on the wall of the heart, for example in the right ventricle with a ventricular septal defect and in the pulmonary artery with a patent ductus arteriosus. Infective emboli pass to other parts of the body producing local signs and symptoms, e.g. splinter haemorrhages. The most common organisms are *Strepto-coccus viridans, Staphylococcus aureus* and *epidermidis*, but almost any organism such as *Rickettsia* and fungi maybe found. Infective endocarditis should never be forgotten when investigat- ing a pyrexia of unknown origin.

Further reading

Jordon, S. C. and Scott, O. (1989). *Heart Disease in Paediatrics*, pp. 265–71. (London; Butterworths)

Marks, M. I. (1985). *Pediatric Infectious Diseases for the Practitioner*, pp. 698–706. (New York, Springer Verlag)

Index